Type 2 Diabetes Cookbook for Beginners

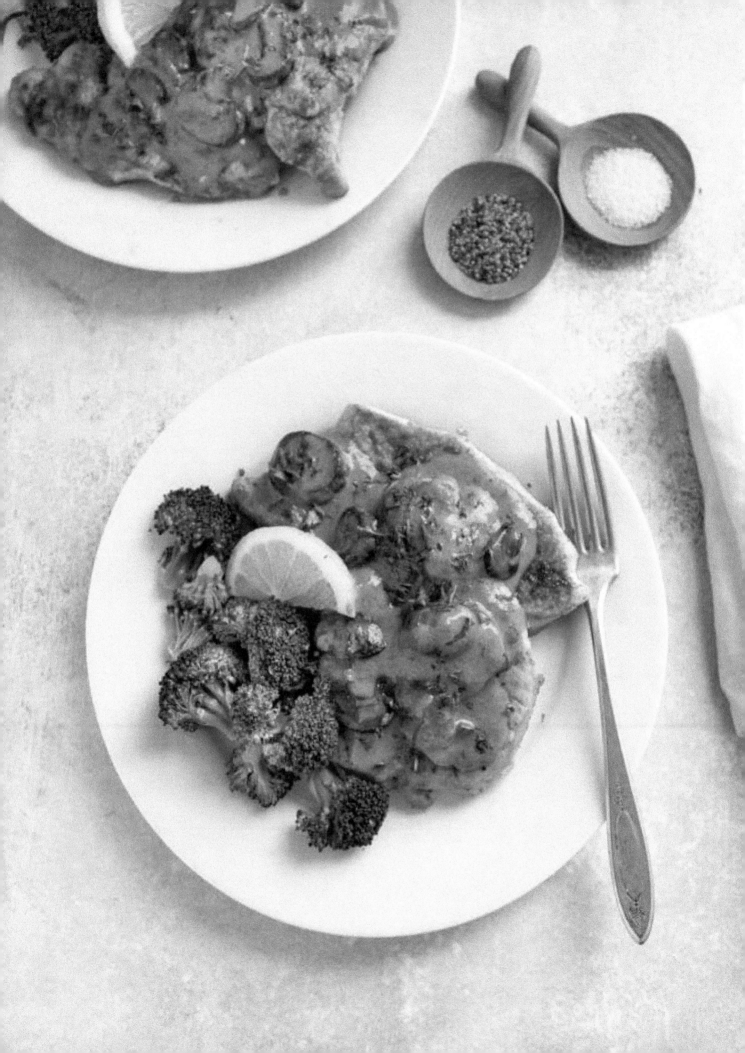

Type 2 Diabetes Cookbook for Beginners

800 Days Healthy and Delicious Diabetic Diet Recipes | A Guide for the New Diagnosed to Eating Well with Type 2 Diabetes and Prediabetes

Jennifer Brown

CONTENT

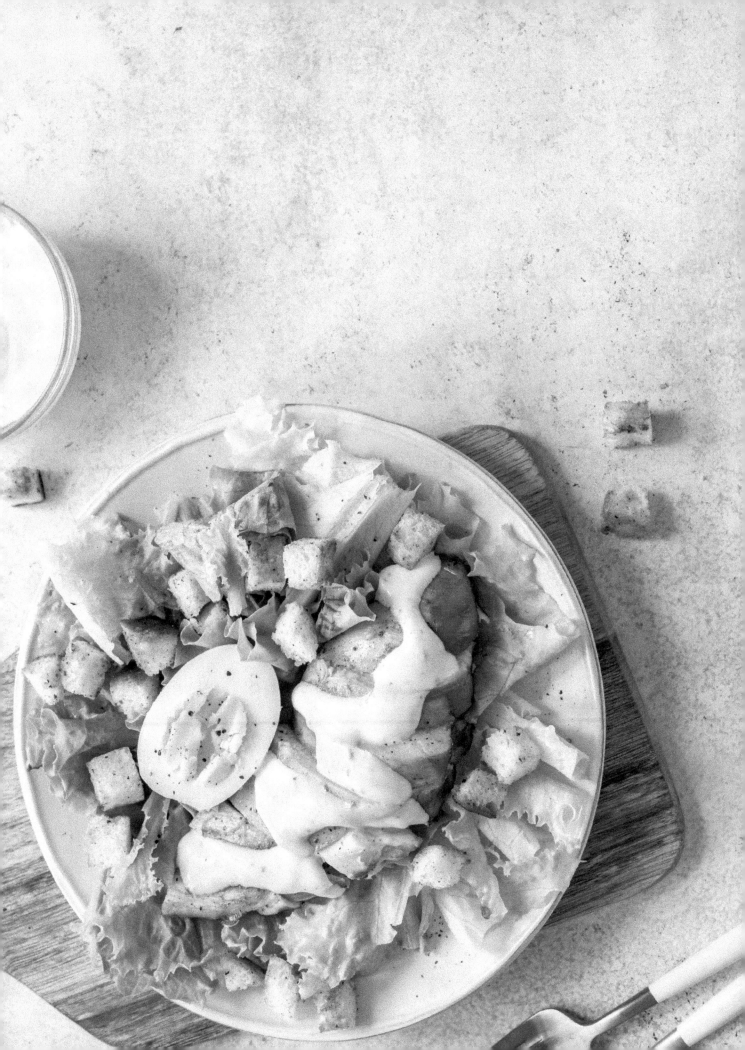

Introduction

A year ago, I was diagnosed with Type 2 diabetes. I was overweight and a total sugar and carb addict. The doctor told me that I would need to be on medication and have to live with this disease for the rest of my life. I watched my father suffer and die from diabetes. I saw him inject insulin every day and I don't want to end up like him. I was worried and became obsessed with finding a cure. So I did my research. I saw many videos and read many books on diabetes, but none of these videos and books gave a simple and straightforward approach to managing diabetes. Due to the lack of simple materials in managing the situation, I did a tremendous amount of research and a realized food management, healthy living, and exercise are the most important factors in type 2 diabetics management.

My simple Type 2 diabetes management method gave me hope. At that point, I committed myself to a strict diet. I did this diet as if my life depended on it. I ate fewer carbohydrates a day and avoided sugar. I checked my blood sugar level at least six times a day to get a complete picture of what everything did to my blood glucose levels. After six weeks, my blood sugar was perfect for a non-diabetic. No medicine. Just diet and exercise. It has now been about ten months. I now do a moderate carb and fat diet. Very little red meat. Fish, chicken, lots of veggies and salads with oil and vinegar, cheeses, and whole grain bread. During winter and I eat pasta, some pizza, and plenty fruit. No sugars. On rare occasions, I eat chocolate. I check my blood glucose levels every morning before breakfast. My blood glucose level never exceeds 5.6 (100). It usually ranges from 4.3 to 5.2, even if I have pasta or pizza at dinner. I do my best to live with as little stress as possible and have a quality sleep.

By following this lifestyle that was extensively built on healthy diet management, I was able to reverse diabetes. I am not alone in this. There are thousands of people who have similar stories. Some people sincerely believe that Type 2 diabetes is an irreversible and progressive disease. They are only repeating what they have been told by the pharmaceutical and medical industries who have a financial interest in not curing diabetes. I am inspired to write this book because of you. The 200 recipes, 21-day meal plan in this cookbook are new alternatives that offer hope and have greatly helped me manage my diabetes, and I believe it will greatly help you too.

Some people are born with diabetes; however, millions of people are diagnosed with Type 2 diabetes every year—otherwise called adult-onset diabetes. Upon diagnosis, if you're like me, you are likely to be upset, confused, and unsure of where to turn. This introductory cookbook is designed to help newly diagnosed Type 2 diabetics patients ease into a new diet and way of living. Type 2 Diabetes Cookbook for Beginners is a must to help you learn. You'll find over 200 helpful recipes as well as advice and general information for living with diabetes. This book is loaded with 21-days delectable meal plan, so in case you're worried you'll have to live the rest of your life eating tasteless food, don't be.

When you're diagnosed with Type 2 diabetes, blood glucose levels are a constant concern. However, with the proper eating routine, you wouldn't have to worry. We all love tasty food; good meatloaf, creamy mac, and cheese or wholesome spaghetti with meatballs. Unfortunately, many people believe

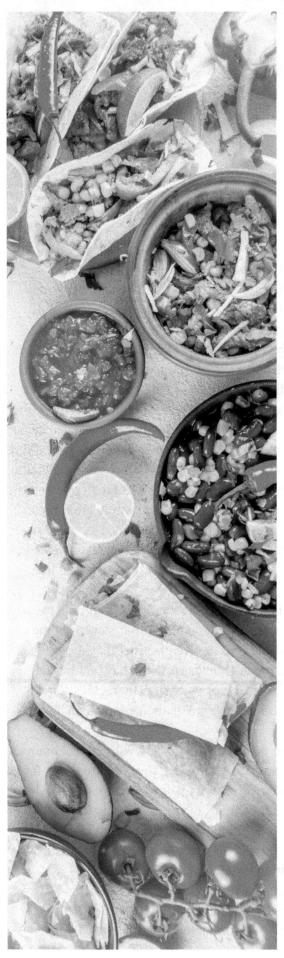

that a diabetes diagnosis means they cannot enjoy these tasty foods. In reality, it only takes some extra care with ingredients and a couple of minor adjustments to recipes to update these tasty foods for a low-glycemic diet. Like every great cookbook, Type 2 Diabetes Cookbook for Beginners is sprinkled with convenient kitchen tips and time-efficient guidance, making it an excellent choice for someone trying to eat more healthily without forfeiting their favorite foods.

This extensive cookbook of diabetes-friendly recipes is designed with love to be perfectly portioned for people with Type 2 diabetes. Regardless of whether you're trying to forestall or control diabetes, your nutritional requirements are almost the same as everyone's. However, you do have to focus on some diet choices, especially carbohydrates. While exercising and living healthy can help, the most important thing you can do is eat healthy. Eating healthy can help you lose a large percentage of your total weight, lower blood pressure, blood sugar, and cholesterol levels. Eating healthier can likewise have a significant impact on mood, energy, and sense of well-being.

Getting diagnosed with diabetes can be terrifying, particularly if you have no idea of the next steps to take. You might start to ask yourself, "Should I be on medicine and supplements? Should I enroll in an exercise program? Should I do this? Should I do that?" These are the thoughts that will run through your mind, and these processes can be overwhelming. However, the most important decision that I made was changing my diet plan. Food is a fundamental part of our survival, and we love to eat. For an individual with diabetes, this doesn't need to change. You don't need to forfeit food for diabetes.

Notwithstanding, exposing yourself to new recipes and meal ideas is never a bad thing. You should simply change your prediabetes favorites into healthier food alternatives. The flavor shouldn't be an issue because there are several ways you can augment your meals to keep them delightful yet healthier. This is where the Type 2 Diabetes Cookbook for Beginners can help. This book will change your eating habits for the better. This cookbook has advice and recipes for all lifestyles, regardless of whether you are battling with portion control or eating out or simply don't have time to prepare a meal every night.

It's significant for individuals with diabetes to monitor their diets intently, as the disease incredibly increases one's risk of heart attack or stroke. This comprehensive cookbook includes snacks and dessert and doesn't forfeit taste for healthy dieting. Sometimes, we all crave for snacks, right?

For most people, meal planning is challenging and tends to be much more challenging for diabetic patients. This cookbook recommends people with diabetes fill their dinner plates with veggies, protein, starch, or grain. All the recipes in the book follow standard basic portioning, allowing you to mix different components of various diet as you wish. This straightforward approach makes the process of building healthy and delicious meals simpler.

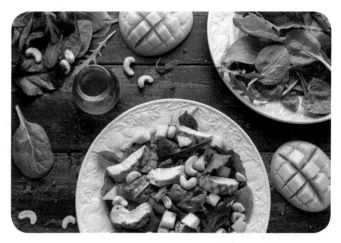

The overall objective of this book is to give hope to Type 2 diabetes patients by helping them manage their condition through the provision of essential information, fundamental skills, resources, and support expected to achieve optimal health. Here's a book that answers the real question about Type 2 diabetes. This book is for recently diagnosed individuals with Type 2 diabetes or anyone ready to control their eating habits. Type 2 diabetics cookbook for beginners is a comprehensive, step-by-step introduction for people with type 2 diabetes. This book guides you through your diabetic journey, encouraging you to make healthy diet choices from the get-go. This book contains a 21-Day delicious and healthy meal plan that supports the quality of life for people with Type 2 diabetes through diet plans while improving the person's personal sense of control and well-being.

The simple recipes used in this book uphold the physiological health of people with type 2 diabetes by maintaining blood glucose as near normal as possible. Diabetes is preventable and can even be reversed. If you're already diagnosed with type 2 diabetes, it's never too late to make a positive change by eating healthier, exercising, and living a healthy lifestyle. Managing diabetes through diet doesn't mean living in deprivation; it means eating a delectable, balanced diet that will improve your mood and boost your energy. You don't resign yourself to a lifetime of tasteless food. This book contains some excellent diabetic diets, with plenty of delicious meals that wouldn't set your blood sugar soaring, helping you prepared to live a happy and well-nourished life despite being a diabetic.

What is Diabetes

Diabetes is one of the leading causes of premature death in the United States. According to records, around 1.4 million new cases of diabetes are diagnosed each year, and an estimated 8 million people are undiagnosed or uninformed of their condition. The estimated number of people above 18 diagnosed and undiagnosed with diabetes is over 30.2 million. Diabetes is a disorder in which the body doesn't use the sugars in food in a typical way. The symptoms of diabetes in people differ, depending on the degree and complexity of the complication. When the body can't get sugar at the required place and time, it prompts elevated blood sugar levels in the circulatory system, leading to complications like nerve, kidney, eye, and cardiovascular disease. Sugar (glucose) is the most preferred fuel for brain cells and muscle. However, it requires insulin to transport the glucose into cells for use. But when insulin levels are low, this means the insulin isn't sufficient to transport the sugar into the cells. This process prompts elevated blood sugar levels. Over the long run, the cells develop insulin resistance, and the attention now changes to the pancreas, which is required to make more insulin to move sugar into the cells; notwithstanding, more sugar is still left in the blood. Due to the pressure on the pancreas, it will eventually "wears out," which means it will no longer secrete enough insulin to move the sugar into the cells for energy.

Without continuous and careful management, diabetes can lead to life-threatening complications, including blindness and foot amputations, heart or kidney disease. It can lead to the development of sugars in the blood, increasing the risk of dangerous health complications, including stroke and heart disease.

What Causes Type 2 Diabetes

The number of cases of Type 2 diabetes is soaring, related to the obesity epidemic. Type 2 diabetes occurs over time and involves problems getting enough sugar (glucose) into the body's cells. Overweight or obese is the greatest risk factor for Type 2 diabetes. However, the risk is higher if the concentration of weight is around the abdomen as opposed to the thighs and hips. The belly fat that surrounds the liver and abdominal organs are closely linked to insulin resistance. Calories obtained from everyday sugary drinks such as energy drinks, soda, coffee drinks, and processed foods like muffins, doughnuts, cereal, and candy could greatly increase the weight around your abdomen. In addition to eating healthy, cutting back on sugary foods can mean a slimmer waistline as well as a lower risk of diabetes.

Symptoms of Type 1&2 Diabetes include:

- Coma
- Confusion
- Blurry vision
- Fatigue or weakness
- Problems having an erection
- Numbness in the hands and feet
- Itching
- Chest pain
- Extreme thirst
- Problems with gums
- Hunger
- Headaches
- Increased urination
- Unexplained weight loss
- Nausea, diarrhea, or constipation

Diabetes is a troublesome disease to live with, regardless of how experienced you are. Adults diagnosed with Type 2 diabetes may have difficulties deciding what to eat and what not to eat. Indeed, even those who have lived with diabetes for quite some time could always use extra guidance and good dieting advice.

Differences Between Type 1 and Type 2 Diabetes

Most people know there are two types of diabetes, but not everyone understands the difference between them. The main difference between the two types of diabetes is that type 1 diabetes, also known as insulin-dependent diabetes, is an autoimmune disorder that often begins in childhood. It is a condition in which the immune system is attacking and destroying the insulin-producing cells in your pancreas, or the pancreas cells are not functioning effectively, leading to a reduction in the production of insulin. Without insulin, the glucose from carbohydrate foods cannot enter the cells. This causes glucose to build up in the blood, leaving your body's cells and tissues starved for energy.

Type 2, also known as adult-onset diabetes, is the most common form of diabetes. Type 2 diabetes is largely diet-related and can be caused by different factors. One factor that may cause this type of diabetes is when the pancreas begins to make less insulin. The second possible cause could be that the body becomes resistant to insulin. This means the pancreas is producing insulin, but the body doesn't use it efficiently. In both type 1 and type 2 diabetes, blood sugar levels can get too high because the body doesn't produce insulin or it does not utilize insulin properly. Diabetes can be managed, and diabetics patients can still live a relatively "normal" life.

How to Prevent Diabetes and Control Sugar Level.

Because type 1 diabetes is generic, blood tests are necessary for diagnosis. However, blood tests that determine the likelihood of type 1 can only be recommended by doctors when a patient begins to show symptoms. An A1C screening tests the blood sugar levels between two to three months and is typically used to diagnose type 1 and type 2 diabetes. Unlike type 1 diabetes which is generic, there are many ways to prevent type 2 diabetes. Ways to prevent type 2 diabetes include:

- Healthy diet
- Quit smoking
- Increase your fiber intake
- Exercise and weight management
- Maintain average blood pressure
- Maintain low alcohol consumption

Treatment for Diabetes.

Type 1 diabetes has no cure; however, it can be managed by injecting insulin into the fatty tissue under the skin. The goal of Type 1 diabetic management is to maintain healthy blood glucose levels before and after meals. The patient needs to understand the required blood glucose requirement and maintain it at all times to experience good health and prevent or delay complications of diabetes.

Different means of injecting insulin include:
- High-pressure air jet injector
- Syringe
- Insulin tub pump

Other measures needed to treat type 1 & 2 diabetes include
- Careful meal planning
- Healthy eating
- Healthy weight management
- Frequent blood sugar test
- Regular exercise
- Medications.
- Glucagon for emergency management of hypoglycemia

Additional Information Regarding Nutritional Goals for Type 2 Diabetic Patients

Carbohydrates

Dietary carbohydrates from vegetables, fruits, beans, starchy foods, cereals, bread, other grain products, legumes, vegetables, fruits, dairy products, and added sugars should provide the largest portion of an individual's energy requirements—both the amount consumed and the source of carbohydrate influence blood glucose and insulin responses. The terms "simple" and "complex" should not be used to classify carbohydrates because they do not help determine the impact of carbohydrates on blood glucose levels. Avoid fruit juices, canned fruits, or dried fruit and eat fresh fruits instead. You may eat fresh vegetables and frozen or canned vegetables.

Protein

Protein is found in poultry, meat, fish, beans, dairy products and some vegetables. Consume more of poultry and fish than red meat and trim extra fat from all meat. Avoid poultry skin. Choose nonfat or reduced-fat dairies, such as cheeses and yogurts. Current proof demonstrates individuals with diabetes have comparative protein prerequisites to those of everybody. Even though protein is important for the stimulation of insulin secretion, excess consumption may add to the pathogenesis of diabetic nephropathy.

Fats

Various studies indicate high-fat weight control diet can weaken glucose resistance and cause atherosclerotic heart disease, dyslipidemia, and obesity. Research likewise shows these equivalent metabolic anomalies are managed or improved by reducing saturated fat intake. Current suggestions on fat intake for everyone apply equally to individuals with diabetes. Reducing the intake of saturated fat by 10% or less and cholesterol intake to 300 mg/d or less. Research proposes monounsaturated fat (like nuts, fish, olive oil, canola oil, seeds, etc) may positively affect fatty oils and glycemic control in certain people with diabetes.

Sugars

In the past, sugar avoidance has been one of the major nutritional advice for people with diabetes. However, research has shown that sugars are an integral part of a healthy diet for diabetes, especially sugar gotten from vegetables, fruits, and dairy products. Added sugars, for example, sugar-sweetened and table sugar products, make up around 10% of the day-to-day energy needs. Refined sucrose gives a lower blood glucose reaction than many refined starches. Foods containing sugars vary in physiological effects and nutritional value. For example, sucrose and squeezed orange juice have comparative blood glucose effects but contain different nutrients and minerals. Consuming whole fruits and fruit juices causes blood glucose concentrations to peak slightly earlier but fall more quickly than consuming a comparable carbohydrate portion of white bread.

The Relationship Between Nutrients and Diabetes

People who have diabetes have excess sugar in their blood. Therefore, managing diabetes means managing your blood sugar level through the consumption of food rich in certain nutrients or through insulin injection. The nutrients in what you eat is connected your overall well-being. The right nutrient choices will help you control your blood sugar level. Eating food reach in the right nutrients is one of the primary things you can do to help control diabetes. There isn't one specific "diabetes diet" for people suffering from diabetes. but a dietician can work with you to design a meal plan to guide you on what kinds of food to eat and what snacks to have at mealtimes. A nutritious diet consists of:

- 20% calories from protein
- 40% - 60% from carbohydrates.
- 30% or lesser calories from fat

Your diet should also be low in salt, cholesterol, and added sugar

Contrary to belief eating some sugar doesn't cause problems for most people who have diabetes. However, it's important to watch the amount of sugar you consume and make sure it's part of a balanced diet.

In general, each meal should have the following nutrients:

- 2 - 5 choices (or up to 60 grams) of carbohydrates
- One choice of protein
- A certain amount of fat

What to Eat

- Healthy nuts fats such as almonds, olive oil, walnuts, cashews and peanuts.
- Fresh fruits, vegetables, and whole fruit.
- High-fiber cereals and slices of bread made from whole grains.
- Fish and shellfish.   • Organic chicken or turkey.
- Protein from eggs, low-fat dairy, beans, and unsweetened yogurt.

What to Avoid

- Processed or fast food, especially those high in sugar.
- Sugary cereals, white bread, refined pasta, or rice.
- Red or processed meat.
- Low-fat products with added sugar, such as fat-free yogurt.

Besides providing diets that will help you manage type 2 diabetes, just like Delicious Dish for Diabetics: Eating Well with Type 2 Diabetes by Robin Ellis, this book offers other benefits as well. The real meat in this book is its use of simple sentences to explain diabetes-related topics such as understand type 2 diabetes, design a menu, how much food should be eaten in a day, food to eat and avoid, and a healthy meal plan for Type 2 diabetes patient. If you are recently diagnosed with Type 2 diabetes, you need a book like this to help get you on the right track for healthy living.

Carbohydrate counting is going to be part of your life now. The recipes in this book are made up of generous amounts of fruits, vegetables, and fiber, which are likely to reduce the risk of cardiovascular diseases and certain types of cancer. The recipes in these book are similar to what you will find in The American Diabetes Association Diabetes Comfort Food Cookbook by Robin Webb, M.S. Embracing a healthy eating plan is the best and fastest way to keep your blood glucose level under control and prevent diabetes complications. Type 2 Diabetics Cookbook for Beginners is here to help you navigate your way around diabetes management by providing a 21-day meal plan made from 200 delicious and healthy recipes to help you develop a good eating habit and ultimately manage your diabetes.

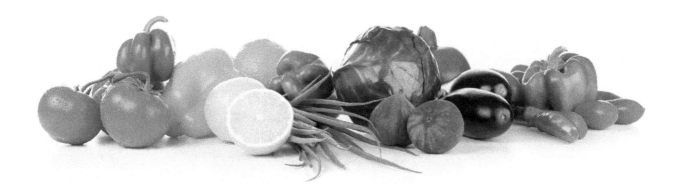

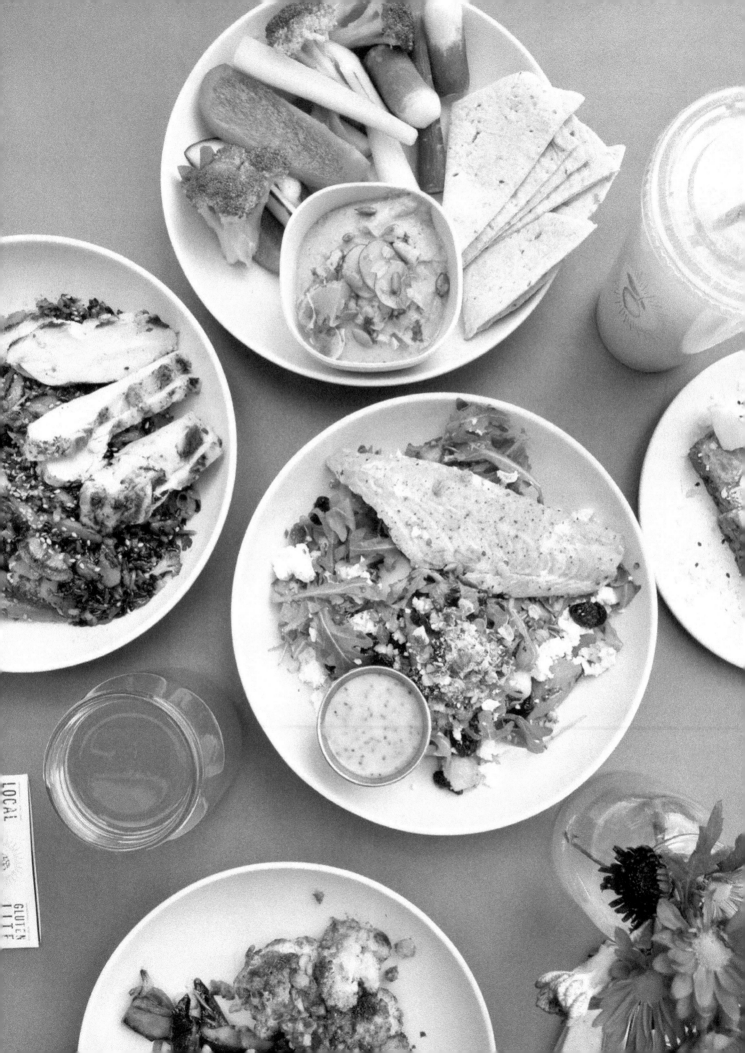

Chapter 1 Breakfasts

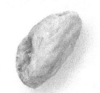

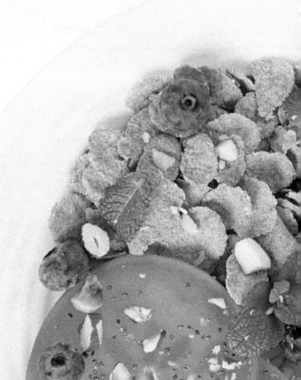

Triple-Berry Oatmeal Muesli

Prep time: 25 minutes | Cook time: 18 to 20 minutes | Serves 6

2¾ cups old-fashioned oats or rolled barley
2 containers (6 ounces / 170-g each) banana
½ cup fresh blueberries
½ cup sliced fresh strawberries

½ cup sliced almonds
crème or French vanilla fat-free yogurt
½ cup fresh raspberries

1. Heat oven to 350°F. On cookie sheet, spread oats and almonds. Bake 18 to 20 minutes, stirring occasionally, until light golden brown; cool 15 minutes. 2. In large bowl, mix yogurt and milk until well blended. Stir in oats, almonds and flaxseed. 3. Divide muesli evenly among 6 bowls. 4. Top each serving with berries.

Per Serving

Calorie: 320 | fat: 10g | protein: 11g | carbs: 46g | sugars: 15g | fiber: 11g | sodium: 65mg

Sunrise Smoothie Bowl

Prep time: 5 minutes | Cook time: 0 minutes | Serves 1

½ cup frozen raspberries
½ large banana
½ cup plain nonfat Greek yogurt
1 tablespoon unsweetened coconut flakes

½ cup frozen strawberries
½ cup cauliflower florets
Water, as needed
2 tablespoons coarsely chopped walnuts

1. In a high-power blender, combine the raspberries, strawberries, banana, cauliflower, and yogurt. Blend the ingredients until they are smooth, adding water as needed to reach the desired consistency. 2. Pour the smoothie into a bowl and top it with the coconut flakes and walnuts.

Per Serving

Calorie: 336 | fat: 14g | protein: 17g | carbs: 44g | sugars: 21g | fiber: 12g | sodium: 69mg

Mi-So Love Avocado Toast

Prep time: 5 minutes | Cook time: 2 minutes | Serves 1

2 slices sprouted grain bread
¼ cup ripe avocado, mashed
A couple pinches of sea salt
Freshly ground black pepper to taste
lettuce or baby spinach

1-1½ teaspoons chickpea miso (or other mild-flavored miso)
Squeeze of lemon juice (about ½ teaspoon)
1 teaspoon nutritional yeast (optional)
2 thick slices ripe tomato, or a handful of chopped

1. Toast the bread. While it's still warm, spread about ½ teaspoon of the miso on each slice. Distribute the avocado over the miso, and add a squeeze of lemon juice and a pinch of salt. 2. Sprinkle on nutritional yeast (if using), and pepper. Top with the sliced tomatoes, lettuce, or spinach.

Per Serving

Calorie: 250 | fat: 8g | protein: 7g | carbs: 38g | sugars: 4g | fiber: 6g | sodium: 1190mg

Coddled Huevos Rancheros

Prep time: 5 minutes | Cook time: 10 minutes | Serves 2

2 teaspoons unsalted butter
4 large eggs
1 cup drained cooked black beans, or two-thirds (15-ounce / 425-g) can black beans, rinsed and drained
Two 7-inch corn or whole-wheat tortillas, warmed
½ cup chunky tomato salsa (such as Pace brand)
2 cups shredded romaine lettuce
1 tablespoon chopped fresh cilantro
2 tablespoons grated Cotija cheese

1. Pour 1 cup water into the Instant Pot and place a long-handled silicone steam rack into the pot. (If you don't have the long-handled rack, use the wire metal steam rack and a homemade sling) 2. Coat each of four (4-ounce / 113-g) ramekins with ½ teaspoon butter. Crack an egg into each ramekin. Place the ramekins on the steam rack in the pot. 3. Secure the lid and set the Pressure Release to Sealing. Select the Steam setting and set the cooking time for 3 minutes at low pressure. (The pot will take about 5 minutes to come up to pressure before the cooking program begins.) 4. While the eggs are cooking, in a small saucepan over low heat, warm the beans for about 5 minutes, stirring occasionally. Cover the saucepan and remove from the heat. (Alternatively, warm the beans in a covered bowl in a microwave for 1 minute. Leave the beans covered until ready to serve.) 5. When the cooking program ends, let the pressure release naturally for 5 minutes, then move the Pressure Release to Venting to release any remaining steam. Open the pot and, wearing heat-resistant mitts, grasp the handles of the steam rack and carefully lift it out of the pot. 6. Place a warmed tortilla on each plate and spoon ½ cup of the beans onto each tortilla. Run a knife around the inside edge of each ramekin to loosen the egg and unmold two eggs onto the beans on each tortilla. Spoon the salsa over the eggs and top with the lettuce, cilantro, and cheese. Serve right away.

Per Serving
Calorie: 112 | fat: 8g | protein: 8g | carbs: 3g | sugars: 0g | fiber: 0g | sodium: 297mg

Breakfast Farro with Berries and Walnuts

Prep time: 8 minutes | Cook time: 10 minutes | Serves 6

1 cup farro, rinsed and drained
¼ teaspoon kosher salt
1 teaspoon ground cinnamon
1½ cups fresh blueberries, raspberries, or strawberries (or a combination)
1 cup unsweetened almond milk
½ teaspoon pure vanilla extract
1 tablespoon pure maple syrup
6 tablespoons chopped walnuts

1. In the electric pressure cooker, combine the farro, almond milk, 1 cup of water, salt, vanilla, cinnamon, and maple syrup. 2. Close and lock the lid. Set the valve to sealing. 3. Cook on high pressure for 10 minutes. 4. When the cooking is complete, allow the pressure to release naturally for 10 minutes, then quick release any remaining pressure. Hit Cancel. 5. Once the pin drops, unlock and remove the lid. 6. Stir the farro. Spoon into bowls and top each serving with ¼ cup of berries and 1 tablespoon of walnuts.

Per Serving
Calorie: 189 | fat: 5g | protein: 5g | carbs: 32g | sugars: 6g | fiber: 3g | sodium: 111mg

Blended Berry Oats

Prep time: 5 minutes | Cook time: 0 minutes | Serves 2

½ cup rolled oats
1 tablespoon ground chia seeds
4 or 5 pitted dates
⅛ teaspoon cinnamon or nutmeg
¼ teaspoon almond extract (optional)
Pinch of sea salt
1 cup + 2-3 tablespoons low-fat nondairy milk
1¼ cups raspberries, fresh or frozen

1. In a blender, combine the oats, chia, dates, cinnamon, almond extract (if using), salt, and 1 cup of the milk. Puree until just combined. Add 1 cup of the raspberries and puree again just to combine. 2. Transfer the mixture to a bowl or jar using a spatula, and stir in the remaining ¼ cup berries. Cover and refrigerate overnight (or for several hours, if eating as a snack). 3. Before eating, add the additional 2 to 3 tablespoons of milk to thin, if desired.

Per Serving
Calorie: 267 | fat: 5g | protein: 8g | carbs: 53g | sugars: 20g | fiber: 16g | sodium: 199mg

Veggie-Stuffed Omelet

Prep time: 15 minutes | Cook time: 10 minutes | Serves 1

1 teaspoon olive or canola oil
2 tablespoons chopped red bell pepper
1 tablespoon chopped onion
¼ cup sliced fresh mushrooms
1 cup loosely packed fresh baby spinach leaves, rinsed
½ cup fat-free egg product or 2 eggs, beaten
1 tablespoon water
Pinch salt
Pinch pepper
1 tablespoon shredded reduced-fat Cheddar cheese

1. In 8-inch nonstick skillet, heat oil over medium-high heat. Add bell pepper, onion and mushrooms to oil. Cook 2 minutes, stirring frequently, until onion is tender. Stir in spinach; continue cooking and stirring just until spinach wilts. Transfer vegetables from pan to small bowl. 2. In medium bowl, beat egg product, water, salt and pepper with fork or whisk until well mixed. Reheat same skillet over medium-high heat. Quickly pour egg mixture into pan. While sliding pan back and forth rapidly over heat, quickly stir with spatula to spread eggs continuously over bottom of pan as they thicken. Let stand over heat a few seconds to lightly brown bottom of omelet. Do not overcook; omelet will continue to cook after folding. 3. Place cooked vegetable mixture over half of omelet; top with cheese. With spatula, fold other half of omelet over vegetables. Gently slide out of pan onto plate. Serve immediately.

Per Serving
Calorie: 140 | fat: 5g | protein: 16g | carbs: 6g | sugars: 3g | fiber: 2g | sodium: 470mg

Rice Breakfast Bake

Prep time: 10 minutes | Cook time: 20 minutes | Serves 4

1¼ cups vanilla low-fat nondairy milk
2½ cups cooked short-grain brown rice
banana (2-2½ medium bananas)
2-3 tablespoons raisins (optional)
½ teaspoon pure vanilla extract
Rounded ⅛ teaspoon sea salt
tigernut flour, for nut-free option)

1 tablespoon ground chia seeds
2 cups sliced ripe (but not overripe)
1 cup chopped apple
1 teaspoon cinnamon
¼ teaspoon freshly grated nutmeg (optional)
2 tablespoons almond meal (or 1 tablespoon
2 tablespoons coconut sugar

1. Preheat the oven to 400°F. 2. In a blender or food processor, combine the milk, ground chia, and 1 cup of the rice. Puree until fairly smooth. In a large bowl, combine the blended mixture, bananas, apple, raisins (if using), cinnamon, vanilla, nutmeg (if using), salt, and the remaining 1½ cups rice. 3. Stir to fully combine. Transfer the mixture to a baking dish (8" × 8" or similar size). In a small bowl, combine the almond meal and sugar, and sprinkle it over the rice mixture. Cover with foil and bake for 15 minutes, then remove the foil and bake for another 5 minutes. Remove, let cool for 5 to 10 minutes, then serve.

Per Serving
Calorie: 334 | fat: 5g | protein: 7g | carbs: 69g | sugars: 22g | fiber: 7g | sodium: 145mg

Potato, Egg and Sausage Frittata

Prep time: 30 minutes | Cook time: 20 minutes | Serves 4

4 frozen soy-protein breakfast sausage links (from 8-ounce / 227-g box), thawed
1 teaspoon olive oil
2 cups frozen country-style shredded hash brown potatoes ,from (30-ounce / 850-g)bag
4 eggs or 8 egg whites
¼ cup fat-free (skim) milk
¼ teaspoon salt
⅛ teaspoon dried basil leaves
⅛ teaspoon dried oregano leaves
1½ cups chopped plum (Roma) tomatoes
½ cup shredded mozzarella and Asiago cheese blend with garlic (2 ounces / 57-××××g)
Pepper, if desired
Chopped green onion, if desired

1. Cut each sausage link into 8 pieces. Coat 10-inch nonstick skillet with oil; heat over medium heat. Add sausage and potatoes; cook 6 to 8 minutes, stirring occasionally, until potatoes are golden brown. 2. In small bowl, beat eggs and milk with fork or whisk until well blended. Pour egg mixture over potato mixture. Cook uncovered over medium-low heat about 5 minutes; as mixture begins to set on bottom and side, gently lift cooked portions with spatula so that thin, uncooked portion can flow to bottom. Cook until eggs are thickened throughout but still moist; avoid constant stirring. 3. Sprinkle salt, basil, oregano, tomatoes and cheese over eggs. Reduce heat to low; cover and cook about 5 minutes or until center is set and cheese is melted. Sprinkle with pepper and green onion.

Per Serving
Calorie: 280 | fat: 12g | protein: 17g | carbs: 26g | sugars: 5g | fiber: 3g | sodium: 590mg

Yogurt Sundae

Prep time: 5 minutes | Cook time: 0 minutes | Serves 1

¾ cup plain nonfat Greek yogurt
¼ cup mixed berries (blueberries, strawberries, blackberries)
2 tablespoons cashew, walnut, or almond pieces
1 tablespoon ground flaxseed
2 fresh mint leaves, shredded

Spoon the yogurt into a small bowl. 2. Top with the berries, nuts, and flaxseed. Garnish with the mint and serve.

Per Serving

calories: 238 | fat: 11g | protein: 21g | carbs: 16g | sugars: 9g | fiber: 4g | sodium: 64mg

Avocado Goat Cheese Toast

Prep time: 5 minutes | Cook time: 10 minutes | Serves 2

2 slices whole-wheat thin-sliced bread	½ avocado
2 tablespoons crumbled goat cheese	Salt, to taste

In a toaster or broiler, toast the bread until browned. 2. Remove the flesh from the avocado. In a medium bowl, use a fork to mash the avocado flesh. Spread it onto the toast. 3. Sprinkle with the goat cheese and season lightly with salt. 4. Add any toppings and serve.

Per Serving

calories: 137 | fat: 6g | protein: 5g | carbs: 18g | sugars: 0g | fiber: 5g | sodium: 195mg

Cinnamon Walnut Granola

Prep time: 10 minutes | Cook time: 30 minutes | Serves 16

4 cups rolled oats	1 cup walnut pieces
½ cup pepitas	¼ teaspoon salt
1 teaspoon ground cinnamon	1 teaspoon ground ginger
½ cup coconut oil, melted	½ cup unsweetened applesauce
1 teaspoon vanilla extract	½ cup dried cherries

Preheat the oven to 350°F (180°C). Line a baking sheet with parchment paper. 2. In a large bowl, toss the oats, walnuts, pepitas, salt, cinnamon, and ginger. 3. In a large measuring cup, combine the coconut oil, applesauce, and vanilla. Pour over the dry mixture and mix well. 4. Transfer the mixture to the prepared baking sheet. Cook for 30 minutes, stirring about halfway through. Remove from the oven and let the granola sit undisturbed until completely cool. Break the granola into pieces, and stir in the dried cherries. 5. Transfer to an airtight container, and store at room temperature for up to 2 weeks.

Per Serving

calories: 224 | fat: 15g | protein: 5g | carbs: 20g | sugars: 5g | fiber: 3g | sodium: 30mg

Chocolate Zucchini Muffins

Prep time: 15 minutes | Cook time: 20 minutes | Serves 12

1½ cups grated zucchini
1 teaspoon ground cinnamon
¼ teaspoon salt
1 teaspoon vanilla extract
½ cup unsweetened applesauce
¼ cup dark chocolate chips

1½ cups rolled oats
2 teaspoons baking powder
1 large egg
¼ cup coconut oil, melted
¼ cup honey

Preheat the oven to 350°F (180°C). Grease the cups of a 12-cup muffin tin or line with paper baking liners. Set aside. 2. Place the zucchini in a colander over the sink to drain. 3. In a blender jar, process the oats until they resemble flour. Transfer to a medium mixing bowl and add the cinnamon, baking powder, and salt. Mix well. 4. In another large mixing bowl, combine the egg, vanilla, coconut oil, applesauce, and honey. Stir to combine. 5. Press the zucchini into the colander, draining any liquids, and add to the wet mixture. 6. Stir the dry mixture into the wet mixture, and mix until no dry spots remain. Fold in the chocolate chips. 7. Transfer the batter to the muffin tin, filling each cup a little over halfway. Cook for 16 to 18 minutes until the muffins are lightly browned and a toothpick inserted in the center comes out clean. 8. Store in an airtight container, refrigerated, for up to 5 days.

Per Serving

calories: 121 | fat: 7g | protein: 2g | carbs: 16g | sugars: 7g | fiber: 2g | sodium: 106mg

Breakfast Egg Bites

Prep time: 10 minutes | Cook time: 25 minutes | Serves 8

Nonstick cooking spray
6 eggs, beaten
¼ cup unsweetened plain almond milk
1 red bell pepper, diced
1 cup chopped spinach
¼ cup crumbled goat cheese
½ cup sliced brown mushrooms
¼ cup sliced sun-dried tomatoes
Salt and freshly ground black pepper, to taste

Preheat the oven to 350°F (180°C). Spray 8 muffin cups of a 12-cup muffin tin with nonstick cooking spray. Set aside. 2. In a large mixing bowl, combine the eggs, almond milk, bell pepper, spinach, goat cheese, mushrooms, and tomatoes. Season with salt and pepper. 3. Fill the prepared muffin cups three-fourths full with the egg mixture. Bake for 20 to 25 minutes until the eggs are set. Let cool slightly and remove the egg bites from the muffin tin. 4. Serve warm, or store in an airtight container in the refrigerator for up to 5 days or in the freezer for up to 1 month.

Per Serving

calories: 68 | fat: 4g | protein: 6g | carbs: 3g | sugars: 2g | fiber: 1g | sodium: 126mg

Carrot Oat Pancakes

Prep time: 10 minutes | Cook time: 20 minutes | Serves 4

1 cup rolled oats
1 cup shredded carrots
1 cup low-fat cottage cheese
2 eggs
½ cup unsweetened plain almond milk
1 teaspoon baking powder
½ teaspoon ground cinnamon
2 tablespoons ground flaxseed
¼ cup plain nonfat Greek yogurt
1 tablespoon pure maple syrup
2 teaspoons canola oil, divided

In a blender jar, process the oats until they resemble flour. Add the carrots, cottage cheese, eggs, almond milk, baking powder, cinnamon, and flaxseed to the jar. Process until smooth. 2. In a small bowl, combine the yogurt and maple syrup and stir well. Set aside. 3. In a large skillet, heat 1 teaspoon of oil over medium heat. Using a measuring cup, add ¼ cup of batter per pancake to the skillet. Cook for 1 to 2 minutes until bubbles form on the surface, and flip the pancakes. Cook for another minute until the pancakes are browned and cooked through. Repeat with the remaining 1 teaspoon of oil and remaining batter. 4. Serve warm topped with the maple yogurt.

Per Serving

calories: 227 | fat: 8g | protein: 14g | carbs: 24g | sugars: 6g | fiber: 4g | sodium: 402mg

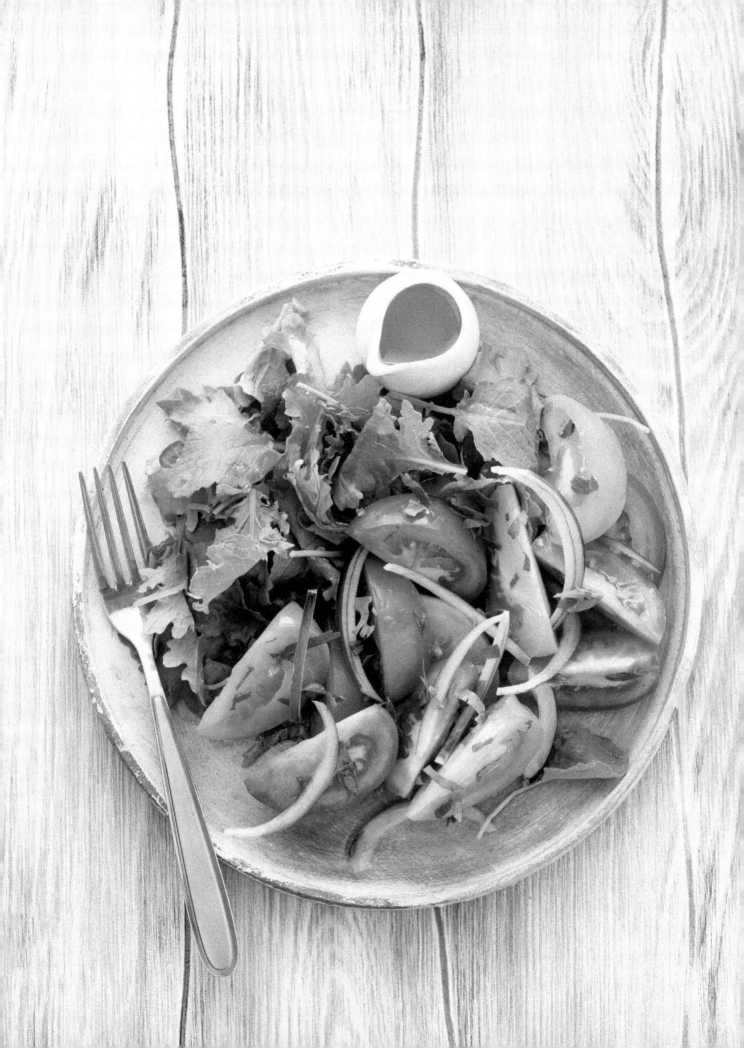

Chapter 2 Meatless Mains

Falafel with Creamy Garlic-Yogurt Sauce

Prep time: 15 minutes | Cook time: 10 minutes | Serves 4

FOR THE SAUCE

¾ cup plain nonfat Greek yogurt

Juice of 1 lemon

¼ teaspoon salt

3 garlic cloves, minced

1 tablespoon extra-virgin olive oil

FOR THE FALAFEL

1 (15-ounce) can low-sodium chickpeas, drained and rinsed

2 tablespoons chopped fresh parsley

¼ teaspoon salt

8 large lettuce leaves, chopped

1 tomato, diced

2 garlic cloves, roughly chopped

2 tablespoons whole-wheat flour

½ teaspoon ground cumin

2 teaspoons canola oil, divided

1 cucumber, chopped

TO MAKE THE SAUCE 1. In a small bowl, combine the yogurt, garlic, lemon juice, olive oil, and salt, and mix well. Cover and refrigerate until ready to serve.

TO MAKE THE FALAFEL 1. In a food processor or blender, combine the chickpeas and garlic, and pulse until chopped well but not creamy. Add the flour, parsley, cumin, and salt. Pulse several more times until incorporated. 2. Using your hands, form the mixture into balls, using about 1 tablespoon of mixture for each ball. 3. In a medium skillet, heat 1 teaspoon of canola oil over medium-high heat. Working in batches, add the falafel to the skillet, cooking on each side for 2 to 3 minutes until browned and crisp. Remove the falafel from the skillet, and repeat with the remaining oil and falafel until all are cooked. 4. Divide the lettuce, cucumber, and tomato among 4 plates. 5. Top each plate with 2 falafel and 2 tablespoons of sauce. Serve immediately.

Per Serving

Calorie: 219 | fat: 8g | protein: 12g | carbs: 27g | sugars: 6g | fiber: 7g | sodium: 462mg

Curried Lentils with Rice

Prep time: 20 minutes | Cook time: 30 minutes | Serves 4

1 tablespoon canola oil

1 cup shredded carrots

2 teaspoons curry powder

¾ cup dried red lentils, sorted, rinsed

½ teaspoon salt

2 teaspoons butter

1 cup coarsely chopped cauliflower

1 large onion, chopped (1 cup)

2½ cups water

½ cup uncooked long-grain rice

1 cup frozen shelled edamame (green soybeans)

¼ cup chopped dry-roasted peanuts

1. In 12-inch nonstick skillet, heat oil over medium-high heat. Add cauliflower, carrots and onion. Cook about 3 minutes, stirring occasionally, until softened. Stir in curry powder; cook and stir 1 minute. 2. Add water; heat to boiling. Stir in lentils, rice and salt; return to boiling. Reduce heat; cover and simmer 12 to 15 minutes or until lentils and rice are almost tender. 3. Stir in edamame; cook uncovered 5 to 10 minutes or until liquid is absorbed and lentils and rice are tender. Gently stir in butter until melted. Just before serving, sprinkle with peanuts.

Per Serving

Calorie: 410 | fat: 13g | protein: 18g | carbs: 54g | sugars: 5g | fiber: 11g | sodium: 430mg

Mushroom Cutlets with Creamy Sauce

Prep time: 15 minutes | Cook time: 20 minutes | Serves 4

FOR THE SAUCE

1 tablespoon extra-virgin olive oil

1½ cups unsweetened plain almond milk

Dash Worcestershire sauce

¼ cup shredded cheddar cheese

2 tablespoons whole-wheat flour

¼ teaspoon salt

Pinch cayenne pepper

FOR THE CUTLETS

2 eggs

1 cup quick oats

¼ cup shredded cheddar cheese

¼ teaspoon freshly ground black pepper

2 cups chopped mushrooms

2 scallions, both white and green parts, chopped

½ teaspoon salt

1 tablespoon extra-virgin olive oil

TO MAKE THE SAUCE 1. In a medium saucepan, heat the oil over medium heat. Add the flour and stir constantly for about 2 minutes until browned. 2. Slowly whisk in the almond milk and bring to a boil. Reduce the heat to low and simmer for 6 to 8 minutes until the sauce thickens. 3. Season with the salt, Worcestershire sauce, and cayenne. Add the cheese and stir until melted. Turn off the heat and cover to keep warm while you make the cutlets.

TO MAKE THE CUTLETS 1. In a large mixing bowl, beat the eggs. Add the mushrooms, oats, scallions, cheese, salt, and pepper. Stir to combine. 2. Using your hands, form the mixture into 8 patties, each about ½ inch thick. 3. In a large skillet, heat the oil over medium-high heat. Cook the patties, in batches if necessary, for 3 minutes per side until crisp and brown. 4. Serve the cutlets warm with sauce drizzled over the top.

Per Serving

Calorie: 261 | fat: 17g | protein: 11g | carbs: 18g | sugars: 2g | fiber: 3g | sodium: 559mg

Homemade Veggie Pizza

Prep time: 15 minutes | Cook time: 25 minutes | Serves 8

Crust

1⅓ cups all-purpose flour

1 teaspoon baking powder

½ teaspoon salt

½ cup fat-free (skim) milk

2 tablespoons olive oil

Topping

1½ cups shredded reduced-fat mozzarella cheese (6 ounces / 170-g)

1 can (14.5 ounces) diced tomatoes, drained

1 cup fresh baby spinach leaves, coarsely chopped

1 cup yellow or green bell pepper strips

¼ teaspoon dried oregano leaves

¼ teaspoon garlic powder

⅛ teaspoon pepper

2 tablespoons freshly shredded Parmesan cheese

1. Heat oven to 400°F. In medium bowl, mix flour, baking powder and salt. Stir in milk and oil until soft dough forms. (If dough is dry, stir in 1 to 2 tablespoons additional milk.) On lightly floured surface, knead dough 10 times. Shape dough into ball. Cover with bowl; let rest 10 minutes. 2. Place dough on ungreased cookie sheet; flatten slightly. Roll out to 12-inch round. Bake 8 minutes. 3. Sprinkle mozzarella cheese over crust; top with remaining topping ingredients. Bake 15 to 20 minutes longer or until crust is light golden brown and cheese begins to brown. Cut into wedges.

Per Serving

Calorie: 190 | fat: 8g | protein: 10g | carbs: 21g | sugars: 3g | fiber: 1g | sodium: 410mg

Italian Veggie Sliders

Prep time: 45 minutes | Cook time: 25 minutes | Serves 6

1½ cups water
½ cup dried red lentils, sorted, rinsed
½ cup uncooked instant brown rice
¾ teaspoon salt
2 tablespoons olive or canola oil
½ cup chopped onion (1 medium)
½ cup finely chopped mushrooms
½ cup chopped red bell pepper
2 cloves garlic, finely chopped
¼ cup finely shredded Parmesan cheese
¼ cup plain bread crumbs
1 teaspoon Italian seasoning
½ teaspoon pepper
1 egg, slightly beaten
12 mini burger buns (about 2½ inches in diameter), split
¼ cup reduced-fat garlic and herb mayonnaise or garlic aioli
⅓ cup packed baby spinach leaves

1. In 2-quart saucepan, heat water, lentils, rice and salt to boiling. Reduce heat; cover and simmer 12 to 15 minutes, stirring occasionally, until lentils are tender but hold their shape and all water is absorbed. Spoon into large bowl; cool 15 minutes. 2. Meanwhile, in 10-inch nonstick skillet, heat 2 teaspoons of the oil over medium heat. Stir in onion, mushrooms, bell pepper and garlic; cook and stir 3 to 4 minutes or until vegetables are tender. 3. Add onion mixture to lentils and rice. Stir in cheese, bread crumbs, Italian seasoning, pepper and egg just until blended. 4. Wipe skillet clean with paper towel. In same skillet, heat 2 teaspoons of the oil over medium heat. Shape lentil mixture into 6 (2½-inch) patties, using about 2 rounded tablespoonfuls for each; place in skillet. Cook 6 to 8 minutes, turning once, until golden brown. Repeat with remaining 2 teaspoons oil and the lentil mixture, making 6 more patties. 5. Place patties on bottom halves of buns. Top each with 1 teaspoon mayonnaise and a few spinach leaves. Cover with top halves of buns.

Per Serving

Calorie: 370 | fat: 13g | protein: 14g | carbs: 49g | sugars: 5g | fiber: 6g | sodium: 650mg

Mozzarella and Artichoke Stuffed Spaghetti Squash

Prep time: 10 minutes | Cook time: 45 minutes | Serves 4

1 small spaghetti squash, halved and seeded
½ cup low-fat cottage cheese
¼ cup shredded mozzarella cheese, divided
2 garlic cloves, minced
1 cup artichoke hearts, chopped
1 cup thinly sliced kale
⅛ teaspoon salt
Pinch freshly ground black pepper

1. Preheat the oven to 400°F. Line a baking sheet with parchment paper. 2. Place the cut squash halves on the prepared baking sheet cut-side down, and roast for 30 to 40 minutes, depending on the size and thickness of the squash, until they are fork-tender. Set aside to cool slightly. 3. In a large bowl, mix the cottage cheese, 2 tablespoons of mozzarella cheese, garlic, artichoke hearts, kale, salt, and pepper. 4. Preheat the broiler to high. 5. Using a fork, break apart the flesh of the spaghetti squash into strands, being careful to leave the skin intact. Add the strands to the cheese and vegetable mixture. Toss gently to combine. 6. Divide the mixture between the two hollowed-out squash halves and top with the remaining 2 tablespoons of cheese. 7. Broil for 5 to 7 minutes until browned and heated through. 8. Cut each piece of stuffed squash in half to serve.

Per Serving
Calorie: 142 | fat: 4g | protein: 9g | carbs: 19g | sugars: 10g | fiber: 4g | sodium: 312mg

Lentil-Corn Burgers

Prep time: 30 minutes | Cook time: 25 minutes | Makes 6 burgers

1½ cups water
1 cup dried brown lentils (8 ounces), sorted, rinsed
¼ teaspoon salt
¾ cup unseasoned bread crumbs
2 teaspoons salt-free southwestern chipotle seasoning
1 can (11 ounces) vacuum-packed whole-kernel corn with red and green peppers, drained
2 eggs, slightly beaten
1 tablespoon canola oil
6 lettuce leaves
6 round 100% whole wheat thin sandwich rolls (4 inch)
3 tablespoons light mayonnaise
6 tomato slices
6 thin onion slices

1. In 2-quart saucepan, heat water, lentils and salt to boiling. Reduce heat; cover and simmer 12 to 15 minutes, stirring occasionally, until lentils are tender yet hold their shape; drain. Spoon into large bowl; cool 15 minutes. 2. Into cooled lentils, lightly stir bread crumbs, seasoning, corn, and eggs. Form mixture into 6 patties about ½ inch thick and 3½ to 4 inches in diameter; place on platter or cookie sheet.

Refrigerate 30 minutes (patties will firm up, making them easier to cook without falling apart). 3. In 12-inch nonstick skillet, heat 1½ teaspoons oil over medium heat. Cook 3 patties 6 to 8 minutes, turning halfway through cooking, until golden brown. Transfer from skillet to heatproof platter; cover and keep warm. Repeat with remaining 1½ teaspoons oil and patties. 4. Place lettuce leaf on bottom half of each roll; top with cooked patty. Spread each with 1½ teaspoons mayonnaise over patty; top with 1 slice tomato, 1 slice onion, and roll top.

Per Serving

Calorie: 370 | fat: 9g | protein: 18g | carbs: 55g | sugars: 9g | fiber: 10g | sodium: 630mg

Falafel Sandwiches with Yogurt Sauce

Prep time: 30 minutes | Cook time: 10 minutes | Makes 8 sandwiches

Sandwiches
¾ cup plus 3 tablespoons water
¼ cup uncooked bulgur
1 can (15 ounces) chickpeas (garbanzo beans), drained, rinsed
¼ cup chopped fresh cilantro
¼ cup sliced green onions (4 medium)
1 tablespoon all-purpose flour
2 teaspoons ground cumin
¾ teaspoon baking powder
½ teaspoon salt
2 cloves garlic, finely chopped
2 tablespoons canola oil
4 pita (pocket) breads (6 inch), cut in half to form pockets
8 slices tomato
16 slices cucumber
Sauce
1 cup plain fat-free yogurt
2 tablespoons chopped fresh mint leaves
¼ teaspoon ground cumin

1. In 1-quart saucepan, heat ¾ cup water to boiling. Stir in bulgur. Remove from heat; cover and let stand about 30 minutes or until tender. Drain; set aside. 2. Meanwhile, in food processor, place beans, cilantro, onions, flour, 3 tablespoons water, the cumin, baking powder, salt and garlic. Cover; process with on/off pulses 10 times or until well blended and coarsely chopped (mixture will be wet). Spoon mixture into large bowl. 3. Stir bulgur into bean mixture. Divide mixture into 8 equal portions, about ¼ cup each; shape each portion into ¼-inch-thick oval patty. 4. In 10-inch nonstick skillet, heat 1 tablespoon of the oil over medium heat. Place 4 patties in skillet; cook 8 minutes, turning once, until golden brown. Transfer patties to platter; cover with foil to keep warm. Repeat with remaining tablespoon oil and 4 patties. 5. Meanwhile, in small bowl, stir together sauce ingredients. Spread 2 tablespoons sauce in each pita pocket. Fill each with 1 tomato slice, 2 cucumber slices and falafel patty.

Per Serving

Calorie: 240 | fat: 5g | protein: 10g | carbs: 39g | sugars: 3g | fiber: 5g | sodium: 370mg

Italian Bean Soup with Greens

Prep time: 20 minutes | Cook time: 45 minutes | Serves 8

2 tablespoons olive oil
2 medium carrots, peeled, sliced (1 cup)
1 large onion, chopped (1 cup)
1 stalk celery, chopped (⅓ cup)
2 cloves garlic, finely chopped
2 cans (15 to 15.5 ounces each) great northern or cannellini (white kidney) beans, drained, rinsed
1 can (28 ounces) diced tomatoes, undrained
2 teaspoons dried basil leaves
1 teaspoon dried oregano leaves
½ teaspoon salt
¼ teaspoon pepper
4 cups vegetable broth
4 cups packed fresh spinach leaves
½ cup shredded Parmesan cheese (2 ounces)

In 5-quart Dutch oven or saucepan, heat oil over medium-high heat. Add carrots, onion, celery and garlic; cook about 5 minutes, stirring frequently, until onion is tender. 2. Stir in beans, tomatoes, basil, oregano, salt, pepper and broth. Cover; simmer 30 to 45 minutes or until vegetables are tender. 3. Increase heat to medium; stir in spinach. Cover; cook 3 to 5 minutes longer or until spinach is wilted. Ladle soup into bowls; top each with cheese.

Per Serving
Calorie: 270 | fat: 6g | protein: 15g | carbs: 39g | sugars: 7g | fiber: 9g | sodium: 990mg

Beet, Goat Cheese, and Walnut Pesto with Zoodles

Prep time: 15 minutes | Cook time: 40 minutes | Serves 2

1 medium red beet, peeled, chopped
3 garlic cloves
2 tablespoons extra-virgin olive oil, plus 2 teaspoons
4 small zucchini
½ cup walnut pieces
½ cup crumbled goat cheese
2 tablespoons freshly squeezed lemon juice
¼ teaspoon salt

Preheat the oven to 375°F. 2. Wrap the chopped beet in a piece of aluminum foil and seal well. Roast for 30 to 40 minutes until fork-tender. 3. Meanwhile, heat a dry skillet over medium-high heat. Toast the walnuts for 5 to 7 minutes until lightly browned and fragrant. 4. Transfer the cooked beets to the bowl of a food processor. Add the toasted walnuts, garlic, goat cheese, 2 tablespoons of olive oil, lemon juice, and salt. Process until smooth. 5. Using a spiralizer or sharp knife, cut the zucchini into thin "noodles." 6. In a large skillet, heat the remaining 2 teaspoons of oil over medium heat. Add the zucchini and toss in the oil. Cook, stirring gently, for 2 to 3 minutes, until the zucchini softens. Toss with the beet pesto and serve warm.

Per Serving
Calorie: 422 | fat: 39g | protein: 8g | carbs: 17g | sugars: 10g | fiber: 6g | sodium: 339mg

Smashed Potato Stew

Prep time: 30 minutes | Cook time: 20 minutes | Serves 6

3½ cups fat-free (skim) milk
3 tablespoons all-purpose flour
1 tablespoon canola oil or butter
1 large onion, finely chopped (1 cup)
4 medium unpeeled potatoes 1½ pound(680 g), cut into ¼-inch pieces
1 teaspoon salt
¼ teaspoon black pepper
⅛ teaspoon ground red pepper (cayenne)
1½ cups shredded reduced-fat sharp Cheddar cheese (6 ounces / 170-g)
⅓ cup reduced-fat sour cream
8 medium green onions, sliced (½ cup)

1. Beat ½ cup of the milk and the flour with whisk until smooth; set aside. Heat oil in 4-quart Dutch oven over medium heat. Cook onion in oil about 2 minutes, stirring occasionally, until tender. Increase heat to high; stir in remaining 3 cups milk. 2. Stir in potatoes, salt, black pepper and red pepper. Heat to boiling; reduce heat. Simmer uncovered 15 to 16 minutes, stirring frequently, until potatoes are tender. 3. Beat in flour mixture with whisk. Cook about 2 minutes, stirring frequently, until thickened; remove from heat. Beat potato mixture with whisk until potatoes are slightly mashed. Stir in cheese, sour cream and green onions.

Per Serving
Calorie: 250 | fat: 6g | protein: 15g | carbs: 34g | sugars: 11g | fiber: 3g | sodium: 740mg

Zoodles with Beet and Walnut Pesto

Prep time: 15 minutes | Cook time: 40 minutes | Serves 2

1 medium red beet, peeled, chopped
3 garlic cloves
2 tablespoons extra-virgin olive oil, plus 2 teaspoons
4 small zucchini
½ cup walnut pieces
½ cup crumbled goat cheese
2 tablespoons freshly squeezed lemon juice
¼ teaspoon salt

Preheat the oven to 375°F (190°C). 2. Wrap the chopped beet in a piece of aluminum foil and seal well. Roast for 30 to 40 minutes until fork-tender. 3. Meanwhile, heat a dry skillet over medium-high heat. Toast the walnuts for 5 to 7 minutes until lightly browned and fragrant. 4. Transfer the cooked beets to the bowl of a food processor. Add the toasted walnuts, garlic, goat cheese, 2 tablespoons of olive oil, lemon juice, and salt. Process until smooth. 5. Using a spiralizer or sharp knife, cut the zucchini into thin "noodles." 6. In a large skillet, heat the remaining 2 teaspoons of oil over medium heat. Add the zucchini and toss in the oil. Cook, stirring gently, for 2 to 3 minutes, until the zucchini softens. Toss with the beet pesto and serve warm.

Per Serving
calories: 422 | fat: 39g | protein: 8g | carbs: 17g | sugars: 10g | fiber: 6g | sodium: 339mg

Caramelized Onion, Potato and Polenta Pizza

Prep time: 30 minutes | Cook time: 50 minutes | Serves 6

Crust
1 cup plus 1 tablespoon yellow cornmeal	¾ cup water
3¼ cups boiling water	1½ teaspoons salt
1 tablespoon olive oil	

Topping
2 tablespoons butter	1 large sweet onion (Maui or Walla Walla),
cut in half, thinly sliced (3 cups)	1 tablespoon sugar
1 cup refrigerated home-style sliced potatoes ,	1 tablespoon olive oil
from (20-ounce / 567-g) bag	⅛ teaspoon salt
⅛ teaspoon pepper	½ cup pizza sauce
1 cup shredded fontina cheese (4- ounces / 113 g)	1 tablespoon chopped fresh oregano

Spray large cookie sheet with cooking spray; sprinkle with 1 tablespoon cornmeal. In 2-quart saucepan, mix 1 cup cornmeal and ¾ cup water. Stir in 3¼ cups boiling water and salt. Cook over medium heat about 4 minutes, stirring constantly, until mixture thickens and boils. 2. Reduce heat; cover and simmer about 10 minutes, stirring occasionally, until very thick. Remove from heat. Stir in olive oil until smooth. Spread hot polenta in 11-inch round on cookie sheet. Cover with plastic wrap; refrigerate at least 1 hour or until very firm. 3. Meanwhile, in 10-inch nonstick skillet, melt butter over medium heat. Add onion and sugar; cook 15 to 20 minutes, stirring frequently, until deep golden brown and caramelized. In 7-inch skillet, cook potatoes in oil as directed on package; season with the salt and pepper. 4. Heat oven to 450°F. Bake crust 20 minutes. Spread pizza sauce over crust; spoon onions evenly over sauce. Top with potatoes and cheese. Bake 8 to 10 minutes longer or until cheese is melted and potatoes are tender. Sprinkle with oregano before serving.

Per Serving
Calorie: 310 | fat: 15g | protein: 8g | carbs: 37g | sugars: 6g | fiber: 3g | sodium: 880mg

Mushroom Pesto Flatbread Pizza

Prep time: 5 minutes | Cook time: 15 minutes | Serves 2

1 teaspoon extra-virgin olive oil	½ cup sliced mushrooms
½ red onion, sliced	Salt and freshly ground black pepper, to taste
¼ cup store-bought pesto sauce	2 whole-wheat flatbreads
¼ cup shredded Mozzarella cheese	

Preheat the oven to 350°F (180°C). 2. In a small skillet, heat the oil over medium heat. Add the mushrooms and onion, and season with salt and pepper. Sauté for 3 to 5 minutes until the onion and mushrooms begin to soften. 3. Spread 2 tablespoons of pesto on each flatbread. 4. Divide the mushroom-onion mixture between the two flatbreads. Top each with 2 tablespoons of cheese. 5. Place the flatbreads on a baking sheet, and bake for 10 to 12 minutes until the cheese is melted and bubbly. Serve warm.

Per Serving
calories: 347 | fat: 23g | protein: 14g | carbs: 28g | sugars: 4g | fiber: 7g | sodium: 791mg

Vegetarian Black Bean Enchilada Skillet

Prep time: 15 minutes | Cook time: 15 minutes | Serves 6

1 tablespoon extra-virgin olive oil
½ onion, chopped
½ red bell pepper, seeded and chopped
½ green bell pepper, seeded and chopped
2 small zucchini, chopped
3 garlic cloves, minced
1 (15-ounce / 425-g) can low-sodium black beans, drained and rinsed
1 (10-ounce / 283-g) can low-sodium enchilada sauce
1 teaspoon ground cumin
¼ teaspoon salt
¼ teaspoon freshly ground black pepper
½ cup shredded Cheddar cheese, divided
2 (6-inch) corn tortillas, cut into strips
Chopped fresh cilantro, for garnish
Plain yogurt, for serving

Heat the broiler to high. 2. In a large oven-safe skillet, heat the oil over medium-high heat. 3. Add the onion, red bell pepper, green bell pepper, zucchini, and garlic to the skillet, and cook for 3 to 5 minutes until the onion softens. 4. Add the black beans, enchilada sauce, cumin, salt, pepper, ¼ cup of cheese, and tortilla strips, and mix together. Top with the remaining ¼ cup of cheese. 5. Put the skillet under the broiler and broil for 5 to 8 minutes until the cheese is melted and bubbly. Garnish with cilantro and serve with yogurt on the side.

Per Serving
calories: 171 | fat: 7g | protein: 8g | carbs: 21g | sugars: 3g | fiber: 7g | sodium: 565mg

Salt-Free No-Soak Beans

Prep time: 2 minutes | Cook time: 25 to 40 minutes | Makes 6 cups

1 pound (454 g) dried beans, rinsed (unsoaked)
5 cups vegetable broth, chicken bone broth, or water
1 tablespoon extra-virgin olive oil

In the electric pressure cooker, combine the beans and broth. Drizzle the oil on top. (The oil will help control the foam produced by the cooking beans.) 2. Close and lock the lid of the pressure cooker. Set the valve to sealing. 3. For black beans, cook on high pressure for 25 minutes. 4. For pinto beans, navy beans, or great northern beans, cook on high pressure for 30 minutes. 5. For cannellini beans, cook on high pressure for 40 minutes. 6. When the cooking is complete, hit Cancel and allow the pressure to release naturally for 20 minutes, then quick release any remaining pressure. 7. Once the pin drops, unlock and remove the lid. 8. Let the beans cool, then pack them into containers and cover with the cooking liquid. Refrigerate for 3 to 5 days or freeze for up to 8 months.

Per Serving (½ cup)
calories: 141 | fat: 2g | protein: 8g | carbs: 24g | sugars: 1g | fiber: 6g | sodium: 5mg

Veggie Fajitas

Prep time: 10 minutes | Cook time: 15 minutes | Serves 4

Guacamole:
2 small avocados pitted and peeled
1 teaspoon freshly squeezed lime juice
¼ teaspoon salt
9 cherry tomatoes, halved
Fajitas:
1 red bell pepper
1 green bell pepper
1 small white onion
Avocado oil cooking spray
1 cup canned low-sodium black beans, drained and rinsed
½ teaspoon ground cumin
¼ teaspoon chili powder
¼ teaspoon garlic powder
4 (6-inch) yellow corn tortillas

Make the Guacamole
In a medium bowl, use a fork to mash the avocados with the lime juice and salt. 2. Gently stir in the cherry tomatoes.

Make the Fajitas
Cut the red bell pepper, green bell pepper, and onion into ½-inch slices. 2. Heat a large skillet over medium heat. When hot, coat the cooking surface with cooking 3. spray. Put the peppers, onion, and beans into the skillet. 4. Add the cumin, chili powder, and garlic powder, and stir. 5. Cover and cook for 15 minutes, stirring halfway through. 6. Divide the fajita mixture equally between the tortillas, and top with guacamole and any preferred garnishes.

Per Serving
calories: 269 | fat: 15g | protein: 8g | carbs: 30g | sugars: 5g | fiber: 11g | sodium: 175mg

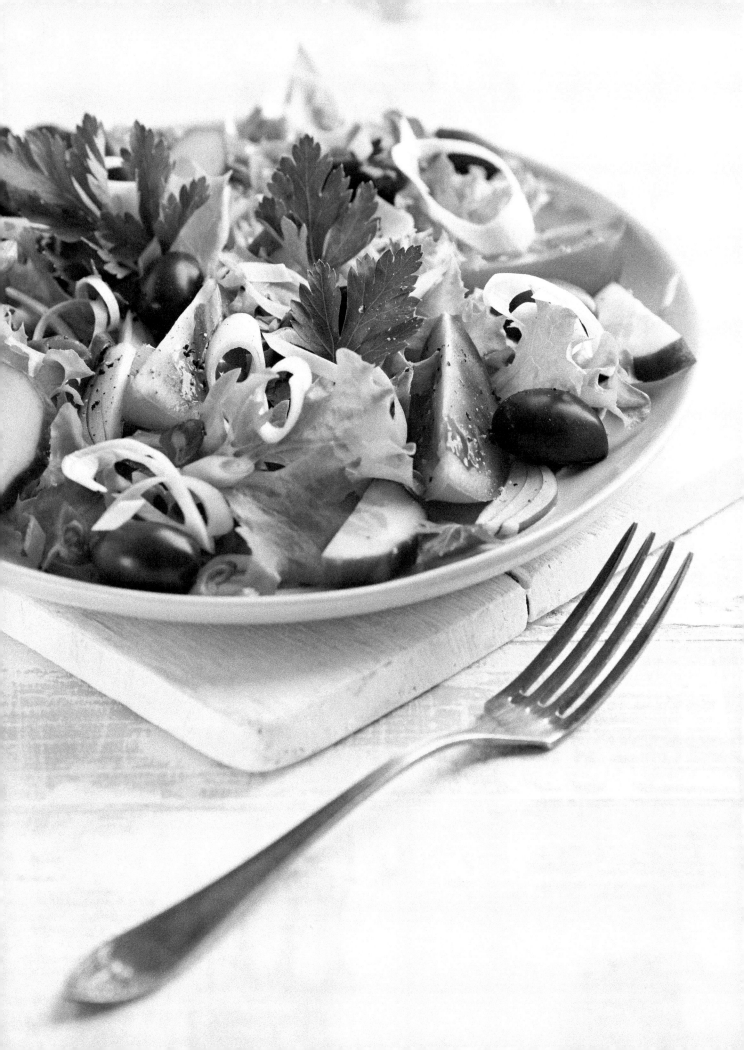

Chapter 3 Vegetables and Sides

Sweet Potato Crisps

Prep time: 10 minutes | Cook time: 30 minutes | Serves 3

1 pound (454 g) sweet potatoes
½ tablespoon balsamic vinegar
½ tablespoon pure maple syrup
Rounded ¼ teaspoon sea salt

1. Preheat the oven to 400°F. Line a large baking sheet with parchment paper. 2. Peel the sweet potatoes, then use the peeler to continue to make sweet potato peelings. (Alternatively, you can push peeled sweet potatoes through a food processor slicing blade.) 3. Transfer the peelings to a large mixing bowl and use your hands to toss with the vinegar and syrup, coating them as evenly as possible. 4. Spread the peelings on the prepared baking sheet, spacing well. Sprinkle with the salt. Bake for 30 minutes, tossing once or twice. The pieces around the edges of the pan can get brown quickly, so move the chips around during baking. 5.Turn off the oven and let the chips sit in the residual heat for 20 minutes, stir again, and let sit for another 15 to 20 minutes, until they crisp up. Remove, and snack!

Per Serving
Calorie: 94 | fat: 0g | protein: 2g | carbs: 22g | sugars: 8g | fiber: 3g | sodium: 326mg

Cheesy Cauli Bake

Prep time: 10 minutes | Cook time: 25 to 30 minutes | Serves 6

3 tablespoons tahini
2 tablespoons nutritional yeast
1 tablespoon lemon juice
½ teaspoon pure maple syrup or agave nectar
½ teaspoon sea salt
½ cup + 1 tablespoon plain nondairy milk
3-3½ cups cauliflower florets, cut or broken in small pieces
Topping
1 tablespoon almond meal or breadcrumbs
½ tablespoon nutritional yeast
Pinch sea salt

1. Preheat the oven to 425°F. Use cooking spray to lightly coat the bottom and sides of an 8" × 8" (or similar size) baking dish. 2. In a small bowl, whisk together the tahini, nutritional yeast, lemon juice, maple syrup or agave nectar, and salt. Gradually whisk in the milk until it all comes together smoothly. In the baking dish, add the cauliflower and pour in the sauce, stir thoroughly to coat the cauliflower. Cover with foil and bake for 25 to 30 minutes, stirring only once, until the cauliflower is tender. 3. In a small bowl, toss together the topping ingredients. Remove the foil from the cauliflower, and sprinkle on the topping. Return to the oven and set oven to broil. Allow to cook for a minute or so until the topping is golden brown. Remove, let sit for a few minutes, then serve.

Per Serving
Calorie: 87 | fat: 5g | protein: 5g | carbs: 7g | sugars: 5g | fiber: 3g | sodium: 270mg

Chipotle Twice-Baked Sweet Potatoes

Prep time: 20 minutes | Cook time: 1 hour | Serves 4

4 small sweet potatoes (about 1¾ pounds)

¼ cup fat-free half-and-half

1 chipotle chile in adobo sauce ,from (7-ounce / 198-g)can, finely chopped

1 teaspoon adobo sauce (from can of chipotle chiles)

½ teaspoon salt

8 teaspoons reduced-fat sour cream

4 teaspoons chopped fresh cilantro

1. Heat oven to 375°F. Gently scrub potatoes but do not peel. Pierce potatoes several times with fork to allow steam to escape while potatoes bake. Bake about 45 minutes or until potatoes are tender when pierced in center with a fork. 2. When potatoes are cool enough to handle, cut lengthwise down through center of potato to within ½ inch of ends and bottom. Carefully scoop out inside, leaving thin shell. In medium bowl, mash potatoes, half-and-half, chile, adobo sauce and salt with potato masher or electric mixer on low speed until light and fluffy. 3. Increase oven temperature to 400°F. In 13×9-inch pan, place potato shells. Divide potato mixture evenly among shells. Bake uncovered 20 minutes or until potato mixture is golden brown and heated through. 4. Just before serving, top each potato with 2 teaspoons sour cream and 1 teaspoon cilantro.

Per Serving

Calorie: 140 | fat: 1g | protein: 3g | carbs: 27g | sugars: 9g | fiber: 4g | sodium: 400mg

Potatoes with Parsley

Prep time: 10 minutes | Cook time: 5 minutes | Serves 4

3 tablespoons margarine, divided

2 pounds (907 g) medium red potatoes (about 2 ounces / 57 g each), halved lengthwise

1 clove garlic, minced

½ teaspoon salt

½ cup low-sodium chicken broth

2 tablespoons chopped fresh parsley

Place 1 tablespoon margarine in the inner pot of the Instant Pot and select Sauté. 2. After margarine is melted, add potatoes, garlic, and salt, stirring well. 3. Sauté 4 minutes, stirring frequently. 4. Add chicken broth and stir well. 5. Seal lid, make sure vent is on sealing, then select Manual for 5 minutes on high pressure. 6. When cooking time is up, manually release the pressure. 7. Strain potatoes, toss with remaining 2 tablespoons margarine and chopped parsley, and serve immediately.

Per Serving

Calorie: 237 | fat: 9g | protein: 5g | carbs: 37g | sugars: 3g | fiber: 4g | sodium: 389mg

Best Brown Rice

Prep time: 5 minutes | Cook time: 22 minutes | Serves 6 to 12

2 cups brown rice
2½ cups water

1. Rinse brown rice in a fine-mesh strainer. 2. Add rice and water to the inner pot of the Instant Pot. 3. Secure the lid and make sure vent is on sealing. 4. Use Manual setting and select 22 minutes cooking time on high pressure. 5. When cooking time is done, let the pressure release naturally for 10 minutes, then press Cancel and manually release any remaining pressure.
Per Serving Calorie: 114 | fat: 1g | protein: 2g | carbs: 23g | sugars: 0g | fiber: 1g | sodium: 3mg

Caramelized Onions

Prep time: 10 minutes | Cook time: 35 minutes | Serves 8

4 tablespoons margarine
6 large Vidalia or other sweet onions, sliced into thin half rings
1(10-ounce / 283-g) can chicken, or vegetable, broth

1. Press Sauté on the Instant Pot. Add in the margarine and let melt. 2. Once the margarine is melted, stir in the onions and sauté for about 5 minutes. Pour in the broth and then press Cancel. 3. Secure the lid and make sure vent is set to sealing. Press Manual and set time for 20 minutes. 4. When cook time is up, release the pressure manually. Remove the lid and press Sauté. Stir the onion mixture for about 10 more minutes, allowing extra liquid to cook off.
Per Serving
Calorie: 123 | fat: 6g | protein: 2g | carbs: 15g | sugars: 10g | fiber: 3g | sodium: 325mg

Peas with Mushrooms and Thyme

Prep time: 10 minutes | Cook time: 10 minutes | Serves 6

2 teaspoons olive, canola or soybean oil
1 medium onion, diced (½ cup)
1 cup sliced fresh mushrooms
1 bag (16 ounces / 454-g) frozen sweet peas
¼ teaspoon coarse (kosher or sea) salt
⅛ teaspoon white pepper
1 teaspoon chopped fresh or ¼ teaspoon dried thyme leaves

In 10-inch skillet, heat oil over medium heat. Add onion and mushrooms; cook 3 minutes, stirring occasionally. Stir in peas. Cook 3 to 5 minutes, stirring occasionally, until vegetables are tender. 2. Sprinkle with salt, pepper and thyme. Serve immediately.
Per Serving
Calorie: 80 | fat: 1g | protein: 4g | carbs: 11g | sugars: 4g | fiber: 2g | sodium: 150mg

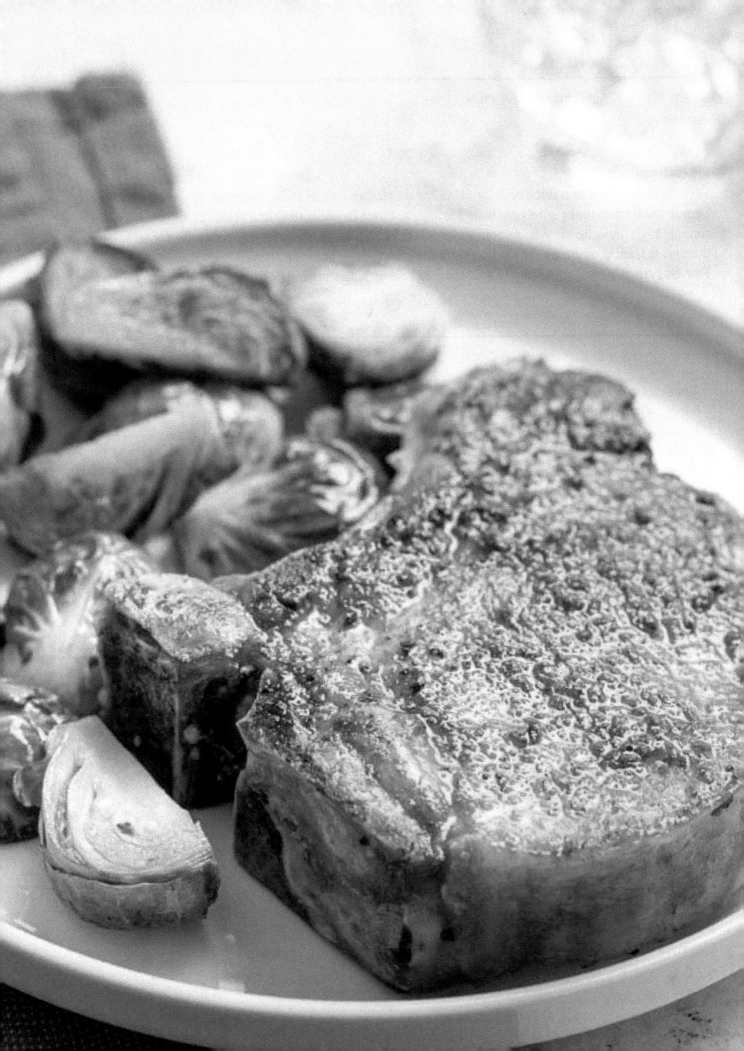

Chapter 4 Beef, Pork, and Lamb

Red Wine Pot Roast with Winter Vegetables

Prep time: 10 minutes | Cook time: 1 hour 35 minutes | Serves 6

1 (3-pound / 1.4 kg) boneless beef chuck roast or bottom round roast (see Note)

2 teaspoons fine sea salt

1 teaspoon freshly ground black pepper

1 tablespoon cold-pressed avocado oil

4 large shallots, quartered

4 garlic cloves, minced

1 cup dry red wine

2 tablespoons Dijon mustard

2 teaspoons chopped fresh rosemary

1 pound (454 g) parsnips or turnips, cut into ½-inch pieces

1 pound (454 g) carrots, cut into ½-inch pieces

4 celery stalks, cut into ½-inch pieces

1. Put the beef onto a plate, pat it dry with paper towels, and then season all over with the salt and pepper. 2. Select the Sauté setting on the Instant Pot and heat the oil for 2 minutes. Using tongs, lower the roast into the pot and sear for about 4 minutes, until browned on the first side. Flip the roast and sear for about 4 minutes more, until browned on the second side. Return the roast to the plate. 3. Add the shallots to the pot and sauté for about 2 minutes, until they begin to soften. Add the garlic and sauté for about 1 minute more. Stir in the wine, mustard, and rosemary, using a wooden spoon to nudge any browned bits from the bottom of the pot. Return the roast to the pot, then spoon some of the cooking liquid over the top. 4. Secure the lid and set the Pressure Release to Sealing. Press the Cancel button to reset the cooking program, then select the Meat/Stew setting and set the cooking time for 1 hour 5 minutes at high pressure. (The pot will take about 5 minutes to come up to pressure before the cooking program begins.) 5. When the cooking program ends, let the pressure release naturally for at least 15 minutes, then move the Pressure Release to Venting to release any remaining steam. Open the pot and, using tongs, carefully transfer the pot roast to a cutting board. Tent with aluminum foil to keep warm. 6. Add the parsnips, carrots, and celery to the pot. 7. Secure the lid and set the Pressure Release to Sealing. Press the Cancel button to reset the cooking program, then select the Pressure Cook or Manual setting and set the cooking time for 3 minutes at low pressure. (The pot will take about 10 minutes to come up to pressure before the cooking program begins.) 8. When the cooking program ends, perform a quick pressure release by moving the Pressure Release to Venting. Open the pot and, using a slotted spoon, transfer the vegetables to a serving dish. Wearing heat-resistant mitts, lift out the inner pot and pour the cooking liquid into a gravy boat or other serving vessel with a spout. (If you like, use a fat separator to remove the fat from the liquid before serving.) 9. If the roast was tied, snip the string and discard. Carve the roast against the grain into ½-inch-thick slices and arrange them on the dish with the vegetables. Pour some cooking liquid over the roast and serve, passing the remaining cooking liquid on the side.

Per Serving

Calorie: 448 | fat: 25g | protein: 26g | carbs: 26g | sugars: 7g | fiber: 6g | sodium: 945mg

Salisbury Steaks with Seared Cauliflower

Prep time: 5 minutes | Cook time: 30 minutes | Serves 4

Salisbury Steaks

1 pound (454 g) 95 percent lean ground beef

1 large egg

¼ teaspoon freshly ground black pepper

1 small yellow onion, sliced

8 ounces cremini or button mushrooms, sliced

2 tablespoons tomato paste

1 cup low-sodium roasted beef bone broth

⅓ cup almond flour

½ teaspoon fine sea salt

2 tablespoons cold-pressed avocado oil

1 garlic clove, chopped

½ teaspoon fine sea salt

1½ teaspoons yellow mustard

Seared Cauliflower

1 tablespoon olive oil

2 tablespoons chopped fresh flat-leaf parsley

2 teaspoons cornstarch

1 head cauliflower, cut into bite-size florets

¼ teaspoon fine sea salt

2 teaspoons water

1. To make the steaks: In a bowl, combine the beef, almond flour, egg, salt, and pepper and mix with your hands until all of the ingredients are evenly distributed. Divide the mixture into four equal portions, then shape each portion into an oval patty about ½ inch thick. 2. Select the Sauté setting on the Instant Pot and heat the oil for 2 minutes. Swirl the oil to coat the bottom of the pot, then add the patties and sear for 3 minutes, until browned on one side. Using a thin, flexible spatula, flip the patties and sear the second side for 2 to 3 minutes, until browned. Transfer the patties to a plate. 3. Add the onion, garlic, mushrooms, and salt to the pot and sauté for 4 minutes, until the onion is translucent and the mushrooms have begun to give up their liquid. Add the tomato paste, mustard, and broth and stir with a wooden spoon, using it to nudge any browned bits from the bottom of the pot. Return the patties to the pot in a single layer and spoon a bit of the sauce over each one. 4. Secure the lid and set the Pressure Release to Sealing. Press the Cancel button to reset the cooking program, then select the Pressure Cook or Manual setting and set the cooking time for 10 minutes at high pressure. (The pot will take about 5 minutes to come up to pressure before the cooking program begins.) 5. When the cooking program ends, let the pressure release naturally for at least 10 minutes, then move the Pressure Release to Venting to release any remaining steam. 6. To make the cauliflower: While the pressure is releasing, in a large skillet over medium heat, warm the oil. Add the cauliflower and stir or toss to coat with the oil, then cook, stirring every minute or two, until lightly browned, about 8 minutes. Turn off the heat, sprinkle in the parsley and salt, and stir to combine. Leave in the skillet, uncovered, to keep warm. 7. Open the pot and, using a slotted spatula, transfer the patties to a serving plate. In a small bowl, stir together the cornstarch and water. Press the Cancel button to reset the cooking program, then select the Sauté setting. When the sauce comes to a simmer, stir in the cornstarch mixture and let the sauce boil for about 1 minute, until thickened. Press the Cancel button to turn off the Instant Pot. 8. Spoon the sauce over the patties. Serve right away, with the cauliflower.

Per Serving

Calorie: 362 | fat: 21g | protein: 33g | carbs: 21g | sugars: 4g | fiber: 6g | sodium: 846mg

Pork Chops Pomodoro

Prep time: 0 minutes | Cook time: 30 minutes | Serves 6

2 pounds (907 g) boneless pork loin chops, each about 5⅓ ounces and ½ inch thick
2 tablespoons extra-virgin olive oil
½ cup low-sodium chicken broth or vegetable broth
2 cups cherry tomatoes
Spiralized zucchini noodles, cooked cauliflower "rice," or cooked whole-grain pasta for serving
Lemon wedges for serving

¾ teaspoon fine sea salt
½ teaspoon freshly ground black pepper
2 garlic cloves, chopped
½ teaspoon Italian seasoning
1 tablespoon capers, drained
2 tablespoons chopped fresh basil or flat-leaf parsley

1. Pat the pork chops dry with paper towels, then season them all over with the salt and pepper. 2. Select the Sauté setting on the Instant Pot and heat 1 tablespoon of the oil for 2 minutes. Swirl the oil to coat the bottom of the pot. Using tongs, add half of the pork chops in a single layer and sear for about 3 minutes, until lightly browned on the first side. Flip the chops and sear for about 3 minutes more, until lightly browned on the second side. Transfer the chops to a plate. Repeat with the remaining 1 tablespoon oil and pork chops. 3. Add the garlic to the pot and sauté for about 1 minute, until bubbling but not browned. Stir in the broth, Italian seasoning, and capers, using a wooden spoon to nudge any browned bits from the bottom of the pot and working quickly so not too much liquid evaporates. Using the tongs, transfer the pork chops to the pot. Add the tomatoes in an even layer on top of the chops. 4. Secure the lid and set the Pressure Release to Sealing. Press the Cancel button to reset the cooking program, then select the Pressure Cook or Manual setting and set the cooking time for 10 minutes at high pressure. (The pot will take about 5 minutes to come up to pressure before the cooking program begins.) 5. When the cooking program ends, let the pressure release naturally for at least 10 minutes, then move the Pressure Release to Venting to release any remaining steam. Open the pot and, using the tongs, transfer the pork chops to a serving dish. 6. Spoon the tomatoes and some of the cooking liquid on top of the pork chops. Sprinkle with the basil and serve right away, with zucchini noodles and lemon wedges on the side.

Per Serving
Calorie: 265 | fat: 13g | protein: 31g | carbs: 3g | sugars: 2g | fiber: 1g | sodium: 460mg

Couscous and Sweet Potatoes with Pork

Prep time: 20 minutes | Cook time: 10 minutes | Serves 5

1¼ cups uncooked couscous
1 medium sweet potato, peeled, cut into julienne strips
2 tablespoons honey

1 pound (454 g) pork tenderloin, thinly sliced
1 cup chunky-style salsa
½ cup water
¼ cup chopped fresh cilantro

1 Cook couscous as directed on package. 2 While couscous is cooking, spray 12-inch skillet with cooking spray. Cook pork in skillet over medium heat 2 to 3 minutes, stirring occasionally, until brown. 3 Stir sweet potato, salsa, water and honey into pork. Heat to boiling; reduce heat to medium. Cover and cook 5 to 6 minutes, stirring occasionally, until potato is tender. Sprinkle with cilantro. Serve pork mixture over couscous.

Per Serving
Calorie: 320 | fat: 4g | protein: 23g | carbs: 48g | sugars: 11g | fiber: 3g | sodium: 420mg

Pork Medallions with Cherry Sauce

Prep time: 25 minutes | Cook time: 6 to 8 minutes | Serves 4

1 pork tenderloin (1 to 1¼ pounds), cut into ½-inch slices
¾ cup cherry preserves
1 tablespoon Dijon mustard
1 clove garlic, finely chopped
½ teaspoon garlic-pepper blend
2 teaspoons olive oil
2 tablespoons chopped shallots
1 tablespoon balsamic vinegar

1 Sprinkle both sides of pork with garlic-pepper blend. 2 In 12-inch skillet, heat 1 teaspoon of the oil over medium-high heat. Add pork; cook 6 to 8 minutes, turning once, until pork is browned and meat thermometer inserted in center reads 145°F. Remove pork from skillet; keep warm. 3 In same skillet, mix remaining teaspoon oil, the preserves, shallots, mustard, vinegar and garlic, scraping any brown bits from bottom of skillet. Heat to boiling. Reduce heat; simmer uncovered 10 minutes or until reduced to about ½ cup. Serve sauce over pork slices.

Per Serving
Calorie: 330 | fat: 7g | protein: 23g | carbs: 44g | sugars: 30g | fiber: 1g | sodium: 170mg

Beef Curry

Prep time: 15 minutes | Cook time: 10 minutes | Serves 6

1 tablespoon extra-virgin olive oil
1 small onion, thinly sliced
2 teaspoons minced fresh ginger
3 garlic cloves, minced
2 teaspoons ground coriander
1 teaspoon ground cumin
1 jalapeño or serrano pepper, slit lengthwise but not all the way through
¼ teaspoon ground turmeric
¼ teaspoon salt
1 pound (454 g) grass-fed sirloin tip steak, top round steak, or top sirloin steak, cut into bite-size pieces
2 tablespoons chopped fresh cilantro

In a large skillet, heat the oil over medium high. 2. Add the onion, and cook for 3 to 5 minutes until browned and softened. Add the ginger and garlic, stirring continuously until fragrant, about 30 seconds. 3. In a small bowl, mix the coriander, cumin, jalapeño, turmeric, and salt. Add the spice mixture to the skillet and stir 4. continuously for 1 minute. Deglaze the skillet with about ¼ cup of water. 5. Add the beef and stir continuously for about 5 minutes until well-browned yet still medium rare. Remove the jalapeño. Serve topped with the cilantro.

Per Serving
calories: 140 | fat: 7g | protein: 18g | carbs: 3g | sugars: 1g | fiber: 1g | sodium: 141mg

Bunless Sloppy Joes

Prep time: 15 minutes | Cook time: 40 minutes | Serves 6

6 small sweet potatoes
1 onion, finely chopped
¼ cup finely chopped mushrooms
3 garlic cloves, minced
1 tablespoon white wine vinegar
2 tablespoons tomato paste

1 pound (454 g) lean ground beef
1 carrot, finely chopped
¼ cup finely chopped red bell pepper
2 teaspoons Worcestershire sauce
1 (15-ounce / 425-g) can low-sodium tomato sauce

Preheat the oven to 400°F (205°C). 2. Place the sweet potatoes in a single layer in a baking dish. Bake for 25 to 40 minutes, depending on the size, until they are soft and cooked through. 3. While the sweet potatoes are baking, in a large skillet, cook the beef over medium heat until it's browned, breaking it apart into small pieces as you stir. 4. Add the onion, carrot, mushrooms, bell pepper, and garlic, and sauté briefly for 1 minute. 5. Stir in the Worcestershire sauce, vinegar, tomato sauce, and tomato paste. Bring to a simmer, reduce the heat, and cook for 5 minutes for the flavors to meld. 6. Scoop ½ cup of the meat mixture on top of each baked potato and serve.

Per Serving

calories: 372 | fat: 19g | protein: 16g | carbs: 34g | sugars: 13g | fiber: 6g | sodium: 161mg

Easy Beef Curry

Prep time: 15 minutes | Cook time: 10 minutes | Serves 6

1 tablespoon extra-virgin olive oil
1 small onion, thinly sliced
2 teaspoons minced fresh ginger
3 garlic cloves, minced
2 teaspoons ground coriander
1 teaspoon ground cumin
1 jalapeño or serrano pepper, slit lengthwise but not all the way through
¼ teaspoon ground turmeric
¼ teaspoon salt
1 pound (454 g) grass-fed sirloin tip steak, top round steak, or top sirloin steak, cut into bite-size pieces
2 tablespoons chopped fresh cilantro

1. In a large skillet, heat the oil over medium high. 2. Add the onion, and cook for 3 to 5 minutes until browned and softened. Add the ginger and garlic, stirring continuously until fragrant, about 30 seconds. 3. In a small bowl, mix the coriander, cumin, jalapeño, turmeric, and salt. Add the spice mixture to the skillet and stir continuously for 1 minute. Deglaze the skillet with about ¼ cup of water. 4. Add the beef and stir continuously for about 5 minutes until well-browned yet still medium rare. Remove the jalapeño. Serve topped with the cilantro.

Per Serving

Calorie: 140 | fat: 7g | protein: 18g | carbs: 3g | sugars: 1g | fiber: 1g | sodium: 141mg

Easy Pot Roast and Vegetables

Prep time: 20 minutes | Cook time: 35 minutes | Serves 6

3-4 pound chuck roast, trimmed of fat and cut into serving-sized chunks
4 medium potatoes, cubed, unpeeled
4 medium carrots, sliced, or 1 pound (454 g) baby carrots
2 celery ribs, sliced thin
1 envelope dry onion soup mix
3 cups water

1. Place the pot roast chunks and vegetables into the Instant Pot along with the potatoes, carrots and celery. 2. Mix together the onion soup mix and water and pour over the contents of the Instant Pot. 3. Secure the lid and make sure the vent is set to sealing. Set the Instant Pot to Manual mode for 35 minutes. Let pressure release naturally when cook time is up.

Per Serving
Calorie: 325 | fat: 8g | protein: 35g | carbs: 26g | sugars: 6g | fiber: 4g | sodium: 560mg

Asian Grilled Beef Salad

Prep time: 15 minutes | Cook time: 15 minutes | Serves 4

Dressing:
¼ cup freshly squeezed lime juice
1 tablespoon low-sodium tamari or gluten-free soy sauce
1 tablespoon extra-virgin olive oil
1 garlic clove, minced
1 teaspoon honey
¼ teaspoon red pepper flakes
Salad:
1 pound (454 g) grass-fed flank steak
¼ teaspoon salt
Pinch freshly ground black pepper
6 cups chopped leaf lettuce
1 cucumber, halved lengthwise and thinly cut into half moons
½ small red onion, sliced
1 carrot, cut into ribbons
¼ cup chopped fresh cilantro

Make the Dressing
In a small bowl, whisk together the lime juice, tamari, olive oil, garlic, honey, and red pepper flakes. Set aside.
Make the Salad
Season the beef on both sides with the salt and pepper. 2. Heat a skillet over high heat until hot. Cook the beef for 3 to 6 minutes per side, depending on preferred doneness. Set aside, tented with aluminum foil, for 10 minutes. 3. In a large bowl, toss the lettuce, cucumber, onion, carrot, and cilantro. 4. Slice the beef thinly against the grain and transfer to the salad bowl. 5. Drizzle with the dressing and toss. Serve.

Per Serving
calories: 231 | fat: 10g | protein: 26g | carbs: 10g | sugars: 4g | fiber: 2g | sodium: 349mg

Mustard Glazed Pork Chops

Prep time: 5 minutes | Cook time: 25 minutes | Serves 4

¼ cup Dijon mustard
2 tablespoons rice vinegar

1 tablespoon pure maple syrup
4 bone-in, thin-cut pork chops

Preheat the oven to 400°F (205°C). 2. In a small saucepan, combine the mustard, maple syrup, and rice vinegar. Stir to mix and bring to a simmer over medium heat. Cook for about 2 minutes until just slightly thickened. 3. In a baking dish, place the pork chops and spoon the sauce over them, flipping to coat. 4. Bake, uncovered, for 18 to 22 minutes until the juices run clear.

Per Serving

calories: 257 | fat: 7g | protein: 39g | carbs: 7g | sugars: 4g | fiber: 0g | sodium: 466mg

Parmesan-Crusted Pork Chops

Prep time: 10 minutes | Cook time: 25 minutes | Serves 4

Nonstick cooking spray
2 tablespoons butter
3 garlic cloves, minced
¼ teaspoon dried thyme

4 bone-in, thin-cut pork chops
½ cup grated Parmesan cheese
¼ teaspoon salt
Freshly ground black pepper, to taste

Preheat the oven to 400°F (205°C). Line a baking sheet with parchment paper and spray with nonstick cooking spray. 2. Arrange the pork chops on the prepared baking sheet so they do not overlap. 3. In a small bowl, combine the butter, cheese, garlic, salt, thyme, and pepper. Press 2 tablespoons of the cheese mixture onto the top of each pork chop. 4. Bake for 18 to 22 minutes until the pork is cooked through and its juices run clear. Set the broiler to high, then broil for 1 to 2 minutes to brown the tops.

Per Serving

calories: 332 | fat: 16g | protein: 44g | carbs: 1g | sugars: 0g | fiber: 0g | sodium: 440mg

Pork Tenderloin Roast with Mango Glaze

Prep time: 10 minutes | Cook time: 20 minutes | Serves 4

1 pound (454 g) boneless pork tenderloin, trimmed of fat
1 teaspoon chopped fresh rosemary
¼ teaspoon salt, divided
1 teaspoon extra-virgin olive oil
2 tablespoons white wine vinegar
1 tablespoon minced fresh ginger

1 teaspoon chopped fresh thyme
¼ teaspoon freshly ground black pepper, divided
1 tablespoon honey
2 tablespoons dry cooking wine
1 cup diced mango

Preheat the oven to 400°F (205°C). 2. Season the tenderloin with the rosemary, thyme, ⅛ teaspoon of salt, and ⅛ teaspoon of pepper. 3. Heat the olive oil in an oven-safe skillet over medium-high heat, and sear the tenderloin until browned on all sides, about 5 minutes total. 4. Transfer the skillet to the oven and roast for 12 to 15 minutes until the pork is cooked through, the juices run clear, and the internal 3. temperature reaches 145°F (63°C). Transfer to a cutting board to rest for 5 minutes. 4. In a small bowl, combine the honey, vinegar, cooking wine, and ginger. In to the same skillet, pour the honey mixture and simmer for 1 minute. Add the mango and toss to coat. Transfer to a blender and purée until smooth. Season with the remaining ⅛ teaspoon of salt and ⅛ teaspoon of pepper. 5. Slice the pork into rounds and serve with the mango sauce.

Per Serving
calories: 182 | fat: 4g | protein: 24g | carbs: 12g | sugars: 10g | fiber: 1g | sodium: 240mg

Curried Pork and Vegetable Skewers

Prep time: 15 minutes | Cook time: 15 minutes | Serves 4

¼ cup plain nonfat Greek yogurt

2 tablespoons curry powder

1 teaspoon garlic powder

1 teaspoon ground turmeric

Zest and juice of 1 lime

¼ teaspoon salt

Pinch freshly ground black pepper

1 pound (454 g) boneless pork tenderloin, cut into bite-size pieces

1 red bell pepper, seeded and cut into 2-inch squares

1 green bell pepper, seeded and cut into 2-inch squares

1 red onion, quartered and split into segments

In a large bowl, mix the yogurt, curry powder, garlic powder, turmeric, lime zest, lime juice, salt, and pepper. 2. Add the pieces of pork tenderloin to the bowl, and stir to coat. Refrigerate for at least 1 hour or as long as 6 hours. 3. Preheat a grill or broiler to medium. 4. Thread the pork pieces, bell peppers, and onions onto skewers. 5. Grill or broil for 12 to 15 minutes, flipping every 3 or 4 minutes, until the pork is cooked through. Serve.

Per Serving
calories: 175 | fat: 3g | protein: 27g | carbs: 10g | sugars: 4g | fiber: 3g | sodium: 188mg

Lamb Burgers with Mushrooms and Cheese

Prep time: 15 minutes | Cook time: 15 minutes | Serves 4

8 ounces (227 g) grass-fed ground lamb

8 ounces (227 g) brown mushrooms, finely chopped

¼ teaspoon salt

¼ teaspoon freshly ground black pepper

¼ cup crumbled goat cheese

1 tablespoon minced fresh basil

In a large mixing bowl, combine the lamb, mushrooms, salt, and pepper, and mix well. 2. In a small bowl, mix the goat cheese and basil. 3. Form the lamb mixture into 4 patties, reserving about ½ cup of the mixture in the bowl. In each patty, make an indentation in the center and fill with 1 tablespoon of the goat cheese mixture. 4. Use the reserved meat mixture to close the burgers. Press the meat firmly to hold together. 5. Heat the barbecue or a large skillet over medium-high heat. Add the burgers and cook for 5 to 7 minutes on each side, until cooked through. Serve.

Per Serving
calories: 173 | fat: 13g | protein: 11g | carbs: 3g | sugars: 1g | fiber: 0g | sodium: 154mg

Cherry-Glazed Lamb Chops

Prep time: 10 minutes | Cook time: 20 minutes | Serves 4

4 (4-ounce / 113-g) lamb chops
¼ teaspoon salt
1 cup frozen cherries, thawed
2 tablespoons orange juice

1½ teaspoons chopped fresh rosemary
¼ teaspoon freshly ground black pepper
¼ cup dry red wine
1 teaspoon extra-virgin olive oil

Season the lamb chops with the rosemary, salt, and pepper. 2. In a small saucepan over medium-low heat, combine the cherries, red wine, and orange juice, and simmer, stirring regularly, until the sauce thickens, 8 to 10 minutes. 3. Heat a large skillet over medium-high heat. When the pan is hot, add the olive oil to lightly coat the bottom. 4. Cook the lamb chops for 3 to 4 minutes on each side until well-browned yet medium rare. 5. Serve, topped with the cherry glaze.

Per Serving
calories: 356 | fat: 27g | protein: 20g | carbs: 6g | sugars: 4g | fiber: 1g | sodium: 199mg

Beef and Butternut Squash Stew

Prep time: 15 minutes | Cook time: 38 minutes | Serves 8

1½ tablespoons smoked paprika
2 teaspoons ground cinnamon
1½ teaspoons kosher salt
1 teaspoon ground ginger
1 teaspoon red pepper flakes
½ teaspoon freshly ground black pepper
2 pounds (907 g) beef shoulder roast, cut into 1-inch cubes
2 tablespoons avocado oil, divided
1 cup low-sodium beef or vegetable broth
1 medium red onion, cut into wedges
8 garlic cloves, minced
1 (28-ounce / 794-g) carton or can no-salt-added diced tomatoes
2 pounds (907 g) butternut squash, peeled and cut into 1-inch pieces
Chopped fresh cilantro or parsley, for serving

In a zip-top bag or medium bowl, combine the paprika, cinnamon, salt, ginger, red pepper, and black pepper. Add the beef and toss to coat. 2. Set the electric pressure cooker to the Sauté setting. When the pot is hot, pour in 1 tablespoon of avocado oil. 3. Add half of the beef to the pot and cook, stirring occasionally, for 3 to 5 minutes or until the beef is no longer pink. Transfer it to a plate, then add the remaining 1 tablespoon of avocado oil and brown the remaining beef. Transfer to the plate. Hit Cancel. 4. Stir in the broth and scrape up any brown bits from the bottom of the pot. Return the beef to the pot and add the onion, garlic, tomatoes and their juices, and squash. Stir well. 5. Close and lock lid of pressure cooker. Set the valve to sealing.Cook on high pressure for 30 minutes. 6. When cooking is complete, hit Cancel. Allow the pressure to release naturally for 10 minutes, then quick release any remaining pressure. 6. Unlock and remove lid. 7. Spoon into serving bowls, sprinkle with cilantro or parsley, and serve.

Per Serving (1½ cups)
calories: 268 | fat: 10g | protein: 25g | carbs: 26g | sugars: 7g | fiber: 7g | sodium: 3887mg

Lamb and Vegetable Stew

Prep time: 10 minutes | Cook time: 3 to 6 hours | Serves 6

1 pound (454 g) boneless lamb stew meat
1 fennel bulb, trimmed and thinly sliced
1 onion, diced
2 cups low-sodium chicken broth
¼ cup dry red wine (optional)
½ teaspoon salt
Chopped fresh parsley, for garnish

1 pound (454 g) turnips, peeled and chopped
10 ounces (283 g) mushrooms, sliced
3 garlic cloves, minced
2 tablespoons tomato paste
1 teaspoon chopped fresh thyme
¼ teaspoon freshly ground black pepper

In a slow cooker, combine the lamb, turnips, fennel, mushrooms, onion, garlic, chicken broth, tomato paste, red wine (if using), thyme, salt, and pepper. 2. Cover and cook on high for 3 hours or on low for 6 hours. When the meat is tender and falling apart, garnish with parsley and serve. 3. If you don't have a slow cooker, in a large pot, heat 2 teaspoons of olive oil over medium heat, and sear the lamb on all sides. Remove from the pot and set aside. 4. Add the turnips, fennel, mushrooms, onion, and garlic to the pot, and cook for 3 to 4 minutes until the vegetables begin to soften. Add the chicken broth, tomato paste, red wine (if using), thyme, salt, pepper, and browned lamb. Bring to a boil, then reduce the heat to low. Simmer for 1½ to 2 hours until the meat is tender. Garnish with parsley and serve.

Per Serving

calories: 303 | fat: 7g | protein: 32g | carbs: 27g | sugars: 7g | fiber: 4g | sodium: 310mg

Corned Beef and Cabbage Soup

Prep time: 15 minutes | Cook time: 26 minutes | Serves 4

2 tablespoons avocado oil
1 small onion, chopped
3 celery stalks, chopped
3 medium carrots, chopped
¼ teaspoon allspice
4 cups chicken bone broth, vegetable broth, low-sodium store-bought beef broth, or water
4 cups sliced green cabbage (about ⅓ medium head)
¾ cup pearled barley
4 ounces (113 g) cooked corned beef, cut into thin strips or chunks
Freshly ground black pepper, to taste

Set the electric pressure cooker to the Sauté setting. When the pot is hot, pour in the avocado oil. 2. Sauté the onion, celery, and carrots for 3 to 5 minutes or until the vegetables begin to soften. Stir in the allspice. Hit Cancel. 3. Stir in the broth, cabbage, and barley. 4. Close and lock the lid of the pressure cooker. Set the valve to sealing. 5. Cook on high pressure for 20 minutes. 6. When the cooking is complete, allow the pressure to release naturally for 10 minutes, then quick release any remaining pressure. Hit Cancel. 6. Once the pin drops, unlock and remove the lid. 7. Stir in the corned beef, season with pepper, and replace the lid. Let the soup sit for about 5 minutes to let the corned beef warm up. 8. Spoon into serving bowls and serve.

Per Serving (1¼ cups)

calories: 321 | fat: 13g | protein: 11g | carbs: 42g | sugars: 7g | fiber: 11g | sodium: 412mg

Sunday Pot Roast

Prep time: 10 minutes | Cook time: 1 hour 45 minutes | Serves 10

1 (3- to 4-pound / 1.4- to 1.8-kg) beef rump roast
2 teaspoons kosher salt, divided
2 tablespoons avocado oil
1 large onion, coarsely chopped (about 1½ cups)
4 large carrots, each cut into 4 pieces
1 tablespoon minced garlic
3 cups low-sodium beef broth
1 teaspoon freshly ground black pepper
1 tablespoon dried parsley
2 tablespoons all-purpose flour

Rub the roast all over with 1 teaspoon of the salt. 2. Set the electric pressure cooker to the Sauté setting. When the pot is hot, pour in the avocado oil. 3. Carefully place the roast in the pot and sear it for 6 to 9 minutes on each side. (You want a dark caramelized crust.) Hit Cancel. 4. Transfer the roast from the pot to a plate.

In order, put the onion, carrots, and garlic in the pot. Place the roast on top of the vegetables along with any juices that accumulated on the plate. 5. In a medium bowl, whisk together the broth, remaining 1 teaspoon of salt, pepper, and parsley. Pour the broth mixture over the roast. 6. Close and lock the lid of the pressure cooker. Set the valve to sealing. 7. Cook on high pressure for 1 hour and 30 minutes. When the cooking is complete, hit Cancel and allow the pressure to release naturally.

Once the pin drops, unlock and remove the lid. 8. Using large slotted spoons, transfer the roast and vegetables to a serving platter while you make the gravy. 9. Using a large spoon or fat separator, remove the fat from the juices in the pot. Set the electric pressure cooker to the Sauté setting and bring the liquid to a boil. 10. In a small bowl, whisk together the flour and 4 tablespoons of water to make a slurry. Pour the slurry into the pot, whisking occasionally, until the gravy is the thickness you like. Season with salt and pepper, if necessary. 11. Serve the meat and carrots with the gravy.

Per Serving
calories: 245 | fat: 10g | protein: 33g | carbs: 6g | sugars: 2g | fiber: 1g | sodium: 397mg

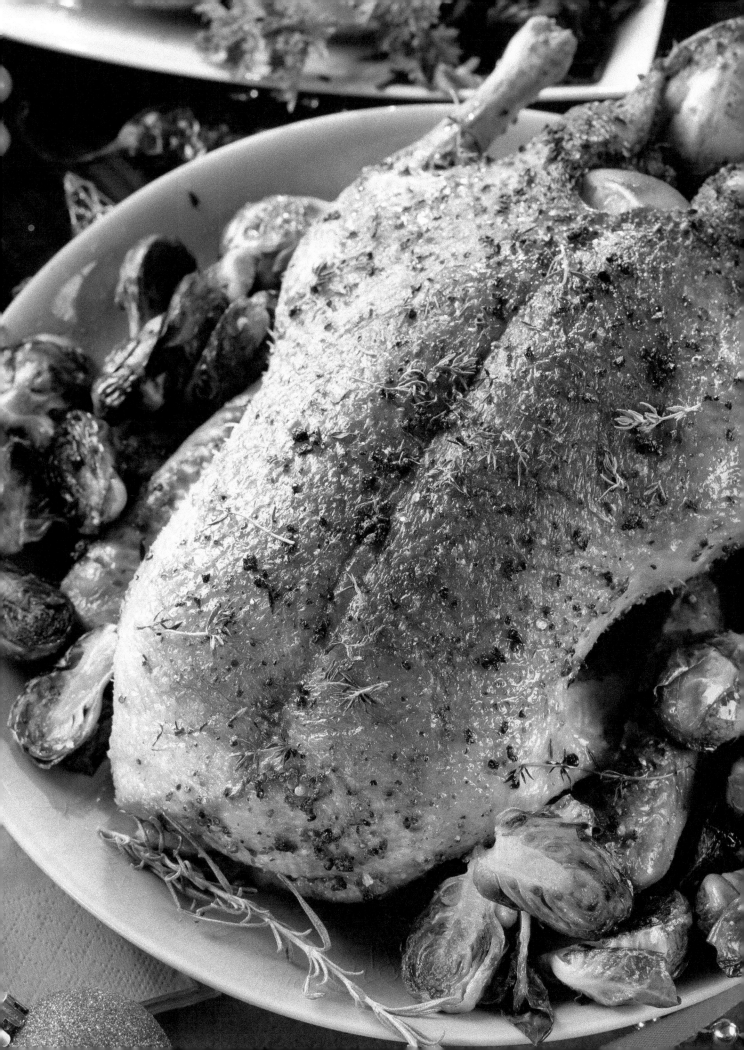

Chapter 5 Poultry

Chicken Caesar Salad

Prep time: 10 minutes | Cook time: 15 minutes | Serves 2

1 garlic clove
Juice of ½ lemon
1 (8-ounce / 227-g) boneless,
skinless chicken breast
2 romaine lettuce hearts, cored and chopped
¼ cup grated Parmesan cheese

½ teaspoon anchovy paste
2 tablespoons extra-virgin olive oil
¼ teaspoon salt
Freshly ground black pepper
1 red bell pepper, seeded and cut into thin strips

1. Preheat the broiler to high. 2. In a blender jar, combine the garlic, anchovy paste, lemon juice, and olive oil. Process until smooth and set aside. 3. Cut the chicken breast lengthwise into two even cutlets of similar thickness. Season the chicken with the salt and pepper, and place on a baking sheet. 4. Broil the chicken for 5 to 7 minutes on each side until cooked through and browned. Cut into thin strips. 5. In a medium mixing bowl, toss the lettuce, bell pepper, and cheese. Add the dressing and toss to coat. Divide the salad between 2 plates and top with the chicken.

Per Serving

Calorie: 292 | fat: 18g | protein: 28g | carbs: 6g | sugars: 3g | fiber: 2g | sodium: 706mg

Mild Chicken Curry with Coconut Milk

Prep time: 10 minutes | Cook time: 14 minutes | Serves 4 to 6

1 large onion, diced
¼ cup coconut oil
½ teaspoon turmeric
¼ teaspoon cinnamon
¼ teaspoon cumin
½ teaspoon salt

6 cloves garlic, crushed
½ teaspoon black pepper
½ teaspoon paprika
¼ teaspoon cloves
¼ teaspoon ginger

1 tablespoon curry powder (more if you like more flavor)
½ teaspoon chili powder
1(24-ounce / 680-g) can of low-sodium diced or crushed tomatoes
13½-ounce can of light coconut milk (I prefer a brand that has no unwanted ingredients, like guar gum or sugar)
4 pounds (1.8 kg) boneless skinless chicken breasts, cut into chunks

1. Sauté onion and garlic in the coconut oil, either with Sauté setting in the inner pot of the Instant Pot or on stove top, then add to pot. 2. Combine spices in a small bowl, then add to the inner pot. 3. Add tomatoes and coconut milk and stir. 4. Add chicken, and stir to coat the pieces with the sauce. 5. Secure the lid and make sure vent is at sealing. Set to Manual mode (or Pressure Cook on newer models) for 14 minutes. 6. Let pressure release naturally (if you're crunched for time, you can do a quick release). 7. Serve with your favorite sides, and enjoy!

Per Serving

Calorie: 535 | fat: 21g | protein: 71g | carbs: 10g | sugars: 5g | fiber: 2g | sodium: 315mg

Greek Chicken

Prep time: 25 minutes | Cook time: 20 minutes | Serves 6

4 potatoes, unpeeled, quartered
2 pounds (907 g) chicken pieces, trimmed of skin and fat
2 large onions, quartered
1 whole bulb garlic, cloves minced
3 teaspoons dried oregano
¾ teaspoons salt
½ teaspoons pepper
1 tablespoon olive oil
1 cup water

1. Place potatoes, chicken, onions, and garlic into the inner pot of the Instant Pot, then sprinkle with seasonings. Top with oil and water. 2. Secure the lid and make sure vent is set to sealing. Cook on Manual mode for 20 minutes. 3. When cook time is over, let the pressure release naturally for 5 minutes, then release the rest manually.

Per Serving
Calorie: 278 | fat: 6g | protein: 27g | carbs: 29g | sugars: 9g | fiber: 4g | sodium: 358mg

Grain-Free Parmesan Chicken

Prep time: 5 minutes | Cook time: 20 minutes | Serves 4

1½ cups (144 g) almond flour
1 tablespoon (3 g) Italian seasoning
½ teaspoon black pepper
½ cup (50 g) grated Parmesan cheese
1 teaspoon garlic powder
2 large eggs
4 (6-ounce / 170-g, ½-inch-thick) boneless, skinless chicken breasts
½ cup (120 ml) no-added-sugar marinara sauce
½ cup (56 g) shredded mozzarella cheese
2 tablespoons minced fresh herbs of choice (optional)

1. Preheat the oven to 375°F (191°C). Line a large, rimmed baking sheet with parchment paper. 2. In a shallow dish, mix together the almond flour, Parmesan cheese, Italian seasoning, garlic powder, and black pepper. In another shallow dish, whisk the eggs. Dip a chicken breast into the egg wash, then gently shake off any extra egg. Dip the chicken breast into the almond flour mixture, coating it well. Place the chicken breast on the prepared baking sheet. Repeat this process with the remaining chicken breasts. 3. Bake the chicken for 15 to 20 minutes, or until the meat is no longer pink in the center. 4. Remove the chicken from the oven and flip each breast. Top each breast with 2 tablespoons (30 ml) of marinara sauce and 2 tablespoons (14 g) of mozzarella cheese. 5. Increase the oven temperature to broil and place the chicken back in the oven. Broil it until the cheese is melted and just starting to brown. Carefully remove the chicken from the oven, top it with the herbs (if using), and let it rest for about 10 minutes before serving.

Per Serving
Calorie: 572 | fat: 32g | protein: 60g | carbs: 13g | sugars: 4g | fiber:5g | sodium: 560mg

Turkey Chili

Prep time: 15 minutes | Cook time: 30 minutes | Serves 6

1 tablespoon extra-virgin olive oil
1 large onion, diced
1 red bell pepper, seeded and diced
2 tablespoons chili powder
1 pound (454 g) lean ground turkey
3 garlic cloves, minced
1 cup chopped celery
1 tablespoon ground cumin
1 (28-ounce / 794-g) can reduced-salt diced tomatoes
1 (15-ounce / 425-g) can low-sodium kidney beans, drained and rinsed
2 cups low-sodium chicken broth
½ teaspoon salt
Shredded cheddar cheese, for serving (optional)

1. In a large pot, heat the oil over medium heat. Add the turkey, onion, and garlic, and cook, stirring regularly, until the turkey is cooked through. 2. Add the bell pepper, celery, chili powder, and cumin. Stir well and continue to cook for 1 minute. 3. Add the tomatoes with their liquid, kidney beans, and chicken broth. Bring to a boil, reduce the heat to low, and simmer for 20 minutes. 4. Season with the salt and serve topped with cheese (if using).

Per Serving
Calorie: 276 | fat: 10g | protein: 23g | carbs: 27g | sugars: 7g | fiber: 8g | sodium: 556mg

Pizza in a Pot

Prep time: 25 minutes | Cook time: 15 minutes | Serves 8

1 pound (454 g) bulk lean sweet Italian turkey sausage, browned and drained
1 (28-ounce / 794-g) can crushed tomatoes
15½-ounce can chili beans
2¼-ounce can sliced black olives, drained
1 medium onion, chopped
1 small green bell pepper, chopped
2 garlic cloves, minced
¼ cup grated Parmesan cheese
1 tablespoon quick-cooking tapioca
1 tablespoon dried basil
1 bay leaf

1. Set the Instant Pot to Sauté, then add the turkey sausage. Sauté until browned. 2. Add the remaining ingredients into the Instant Pot and stir. 3. Secure the lid and make sure the vent is set to sealing. Cook on Manual for 15 minutes. 4. When cook time is up, let the pressure release naturally for 5 minutes then perform a quick release. Discard bay leaf.

Per Serving
Calorie: 251 | fat: 10g | protein: 18g | carbs: 23g | sugars: 8g | fiber: 3g | sodium: 936mg

Baked Coconut Chicken Tenders

Prep time: 10 minutes | Cook time: 20 minutes | Serves 6

4 chicken breasts, each cut lengthwise into 3 strips
¼ teaspoon freshly ground black pepper
2 eggs, beaten
1 cup unsweetened coconut flakes
½ teaspoon salt
½ cup coconut flour
2 tablespoons unsweetened plain almond milk

Preheat the oven to 400°F (205°C). Line a baking sheet with parchment paper. Season the chicken pieces with the salt and pepper. 2. Place the coconut flour in a small bowl. In another bowl, mix the eggs with the almond milk. Spread the coconut flakes on a plate. 3. One by one, roll the chicken pieces in the flour, then dip the floured chicken in the egg mixture and shake off any excess. Roll in the coconut flakes and transfer to the prepared baking sheet. 4. Bake for 15 to 20 minutes, flipping once halfway through, until cooked through and browned.

Per Serving
calories: 216 | fat: 13g | protein: 20g | carbs: 9g | sugars: 2g | fiber: 6g | sodium: 346mg

Savory Rubbed Roast Chicken

Prep time: 10 minutes | Cook time: 35 minutes | Serves 6

1 teaspoon ground paprika
½ teaspoon ground coriander
½ teaspoon salt
6 chicken legs
1 teaspoon garlic powder
½ teaspoon ground cumin
¼ teaspoon ground cayenne pepper
1 teaspoon extra-virgin olive oil

Preheat the oven to 400°F (205°C). 2. In a small bowl, combine the paprika, garlic powder, coriander, cumin, salt, and cayenne pepper. Rub the chicken legs all over with the spices. 3. In an ovenproof skillet, heat the oil over medium heat. Sear the chicken for 8 to 10 minutes on each side until the skin browns and becomes crisp. 4. Transfer the skillet to the oven and continue to cook for 10 to 15 minutes until the chicken is cooked through and its juices run clear.

Per Serving
calories: 276 | fat: 16g | protein: 30g | carbs: 1g | sugars: 0g | fiber: 0g | sodium: 256mg

Saffron Chicken

Prep time: 10 minutes | Cook time: 10 minutes | Serves 4

Pinch saffron (3 or 4 threads)
2 tablespoons water
3 garlic cloves, minced
Juice of ½ lemon
1 pound (454 g) boneless, skinless chicken breasts, cut into 2-inch strips
1 tablespoon extra-virgin olive oil
½ cup plain nonfat yogurt
½ onion, chopped
2 tablespoons chopped fresh cilantro
½ teaspoon salt

In a blender jar, combine the saffron, yogurt, water, onion, garlic, cilantro, lemon juice, and salt. Pulse to blend. 2. In a large mixing bowl, combine the chicken and the yogurt sauce, and stir to coat. Cover and

refrigerate for at least 1 hour or up to overnight. 3. In a large skillet, heat the oil over medium heat. Add the chicken pieces, shaking off any excess marinade. Discard the marinade. Cook the chicken pieces on each side for 5 minutes, flipping once, until cooked through and golden brown.
Per Serving
calories: 155 | fat: 5g | protein: 26g | carbs: 3g | sugars: 1g | fiber: 0g | sodium: 501mg

Chicken with Spiced Sesame Sauce

Prep time: 20 minutes | Cook time: 8 minutes | Serves 5

2 tablespoons tahini (sesame sauce)
1 tablespoon low-sodium soy sauce
1 teaspoon red wine vinegar
1 teaspoon shredded ginger root (Microplane works best)
2 pounds (907 g) chicken breast, chopped into 8 portions

¼ cup water
¼ cup chopped onion
2 teaspoons minced garlic

1. Place first seven ingredients in bottom of the inner pot of the Instant Pot. 2. Add coarsely chopped chicken on top. 3. Secure the lid and make sure vent is at sealing. Set for 8 minutes using Manual setting. When cook time is up, let the pressure release naturally for 10 minutes, then perform a quick release. 4. Remove ingredients and shred chicken with fork. Combine with other ingredients in pot for a tasty sandwich filling or sauce.
Per Serving
Calorie: 215 | fat: 7g | protein: 35g | carbs: 2g | sugars: 0g | fiber: 0g | sodium: 178mg

Sesame Chicken Soba Noodles

Prep time: 10 minutes | Cook time: 15 minutes | Serves 6

8 ounces (227 g) soba noodles
2 boneless, skinless chicken breasts, halved lengthwise
¼ cup tahini
2 tablespoons rice vinegar
1 tablespoon reduced-sodium gluten-free soy sauce or tamari
1 teaspoon toasted sesame oil
1 (1-inch) piece fresh ginger, finely grated
⅓ cup water
1 large cucumber, seeded and diced
1 scallions bunch, green parts only, cut into 1-inch segments
1 tablespoon sesame seeds

Preheat the broiler to high. 2. Bring a large pot of water to a boil. Add the noodles and cook until tender, according to the package directions. Drain and rinse the noodles in cool water. 3. On a baking sheet, arrange the chicken in a single layer. Broil for 5 to 7 minutes on each side, depending on the thickness, until the chicken is cooked through and its juices run clear. Use two forks to shred the chicken. 4. In a small bowl, combine the tahini, rice vinegar, soy sauce, sesame oil, ginger, and water. Whisk to combine. 5. In a large bowl, toss the shredded chicken, noodles, cucumber, and scallions. Pour the tahini sauce over the noodles and toss to combine. Served sprinkled with the sesame seeds.
Per Serving
calories: 251 | fat: 8g | protein: 16g | carbs: 35g | sugars: 2g | fiber: 2g | sodium: 482mg

Chicken Satay with Peanut Sauce

Prep time: 20 minutes | Cook time: 10 minutes | Serves 8

Peanut Sauce:
1 cup natural peanut butter
2 tablespoons low-sodium tamari or gluten-free soy sauce
1 teaspoon red chili paste
1 tablespoon honey
Juice of 2 limes
½ cup hot water
Chicken:
2 pounds (907 g) boneless, skinless chicken thighs, trimmed of fat and cut into 1-inch pieces
½ cup plain nonfat Greek yogurt
2 garlic cloves, minced
1 teaspoon minced fresh ginger
½ onion, coarsely chopped
1½ teaspoons ground coriander
2 teaspoons ground cumin
½ teaspoon salt
1 teaspoon extra-virgin olive oil
Lettuce leaves, for serving

Make the Peanut Sauce
In a medium mixing bowl, combine the peanut butter, tamari, chili paste, honey, lime juice, and hot water. Mix until smooth. Set aside.
Make the Chicken
In a large mixing bowl, combine the chicken, yogurt, garlic, ginger, onion, coriander, cumin, and salt, and mix well. 2. Cover and marinate in the refrigerator for at least 2 hours. 3. Thread the chicken pieces onto bamboo skewers. In a grill pan or large skillet, heat the oil. Cook the skewers for 3 to 5 minutes on each side until the pieces are cooked through. 4. Remove the chicken from the skewers and place a few pieces on each lettuce leaf. Drizzle with the peanut sauce and serve.
Per Serving
calories: 386 | fat: 26g | protein: 30g | carbs: 14g | sugars: 6g | fiber: 2g | sodium: 442mg

Teriyaki Meatballs

Prep time: 20 minutes | Cook time: 20 minutes | Serves 6

1 pound (454 g) lean ground turkey
¼ cup finely chopped scallions, both white and green parts
1 egg
2 garlic cloves, minced
1 teaspoon grated fresh ginger
2 tablespoons reduced-sodium tamari or gluten-free soy sauce
1 tablespoon honey
2 teaspoons mirin
1 teaspoon toasted sesame oil

Preheat the oven to 400ºF (205ºC). Line a baking sheet with parchment paper. 2. In a large mixing bowl, combine the turkey, scallions, egg, garlic, ginger, tamari, honey, mirin, and sesame oil. Mix well. 3. Using your hands, form the meat mixture into balls about the size of a tablespoon. Arrange on the prepared baking sheet. 4. Bake for 10 minutes, flip with a spatula, and continue baking for an additional 10 minutes until the meatballs are cooked through.

Per Serving

calories: 153 | fat: 8g | protein: 16g | carbs: 5g | sugars: 4g | fiber: 0g | sodium: 270mg

Chicken Cacciatore

Prep time: 10 minutes | Cook time: 45 minutes | Serves 6

3 teaspoons extra-virgin olive oil, divided

6 chicken legs

8 ounces (227 g) brown mushrooms

1 large onion, sliced

1 red bell pepper, seeded and cut into strips

3 garlic cloves, minced

½ cup dry red wine

1 (28-ounce / 794-g) can whole tomatoes, drained

1 thyme sprig

1 rosemary sprig

½ teaspoon salt

¼ teaspoon freshly ground black pepper

¼ cup water

Preheat the oven to 350ºF (180ºC). 2. In a Dutch oven (or any oven-safe covered pot), heat 2 teaspoons of oil over medium-high heat. Sear the chicken on all sides until browned. Remove and set aside. 3. Heat the remaining 1 teaspoon of oil in the Dutch oven and sauté the mushrooms for 3 to 5 minutes until they brown and begin to release their water. Add the onion, bell pepper, and garlic, and mix together with the mushrooms. Cook an additional 3 to 5 minutes until the onion begins to soften. 4. Add the red wine and deglaze the pot. Bring to a simmer. Add the tomatoes, breaking them into pieces with a spoon. Add the thyme, rosemary, salt, and pepper to the pot and mix well. 5. Add the water, then nestle the cooked chicken, along with any juices that have accumulated, in the vegetables. 6. Transfer the pot to the oven. Cook for 30 minutes until the chicken is cooked through and its juices run clear. Remove the thyme and rosemary sprigs and serve.

Per Serving

calories: 257 | fat: 11g | protein: 28g | carbs: 11g | sugars: 6g | fiber: 2g | sodium: 398mg

Turkey Meatloaf Muffins

Prep time: 10 minutes | Cook time: 35 minutes | Serves 12

Nonstick cooking spray
1 pound (454 g) lean ground turkey
1 red bell pepper, seeded and finely chopped
3 garlic cloves, minced
½ teaspoon freshly ground black pepper

½ cup old-fashioned oats
½ cup finely chopped onion
2 eggs
1 teaspoon salt

Preheat the oven to 375°F (190°C). Lightly spray a 12-cup muffin tin with nonstick cooking spray. 2. In a blender, process the oats until they become flour. 3. In a large mixing bowl, combine the oat flour, turkey, onion, bell pepper, eggs, and garlic. Mix well and season with the salt and pepper. 4. Using an ice cream scoop, transfer a ¼-cup portion of the meat mixture to each muffin cup. 5. Bake for 30 to 35 minutes until the muffins are cooked through. 6. Slide a knife along the outside of each cup to loosen the muffins and remove. Serve warm.

Per Serving

calories: 89 | fat: 4g | protein: 9g | carbs: 4g | sugars: 4g | fiber: 1g | sodium: 203mg

Brown Mushroom Stuffed Turkey Breast

Prep time: 10 minutes | Cook time: 1 hour 5 minutes | Serves 8

2 tablespoons extra-virgin olive oil, divided
8 ounces (227 g) brown mushrooms, finely chopped
2 garlic cloves, minced
½ teaspoon salt, divided
¼ teaspoon freshly ground black pepper, divided
2 tablespoons chopped fresh sage
1 boneless, skinless turkey breast (about 3 pounds / 1.4 kg), butterflied

Preheat the oven to 375°F (190°C). 2. In a large skillet, heat 1 tablespoon of oil over medium heat. Add the mushrooms and cook for 4 to 5 minutes, stirring regularly, until most of the liquid has evaporated from the pan. Add the garlic, ¼ teaspoon of salt, and ⅛ teaspoon of pepper, and continue to cook for an additional minute. Add the sage to the pan, cook for 1 minute, and remove the pan from the heat. 3. On a clean work surface, lay the turkey breast flat. Use a kitchen mallet to pound the breast to an even 1-inch thickness throughout. 4. Spread the mushroom-sage mixture on the turkey breast, leaving a 1-inch border around the edges. Roll the breast tightly into a log. 5. Using kitchen twine, tie the breast two or three times around to hold it together. Rub the remaining 1 tablespoon of oil over the turkey breast. Season with the remaining ¼ teaspoon of salt and ⅛ teaspoon of pepper. 6. Transfer to a roasting pan and roast for 50 to 60 minutes, until the juices run clear, the meat is cooked through, and the internal temperature reaches 180°F (82°C). 7. Let rest for 5 minutes. Cut off the twine, slice, and serve.

Per Serving

calories: 232 | fat: 6g | protein: 41g | carbs: 2g | sugars: 0g | fiber: 0g | sodium: 320mg

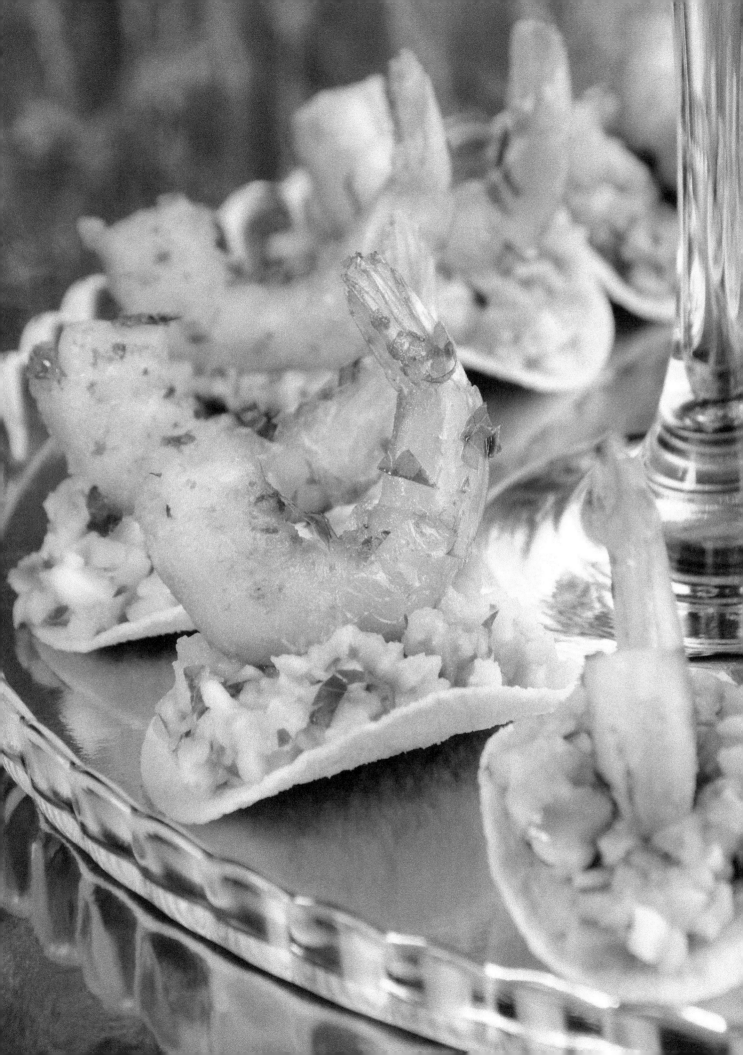

Chapter 6 Fish and Seafood

Tomato Bun Tuna Melts

Prep time: 5 minutes | Cook time: 5 minutes | Serves 2

1 (5-ounce / 142-g) can chunk light tuna packed in water, drained
2 tablespoons plain nonfat Greek yogurt
2 teaspoons freshly squeezed lemon juice
2 tablespoons finely chopped celery
1 tablespoon finely chopped red onion
Pinch cayenne pepper
1 large tomato, cut into ¾-inch-thick rounds
½ cup shredded Cheddar cheese

Preheat the broiler to high. 2. In a medium bowl, combine the tuna, yogurt, lemon juice, celery, red onion, and cayenne pepper. Stir well. 3. Arrange the tomato slices on a baking sheet. Top each with some tuna salad and Cheddar cheese. 4. Broil for 3 to 4 minutes until the cheese is melted and bubbly. Serve.

Per Serving

calories: 243 | fat: 10g | protein: 30g | carbs: 7g | sugars: 2g | fiber: 1g | sodium: 444mg

Honey Ginger Glazed Salmon with Broccoli

Prep time: 10 minutes | Cook time: 15 minutes | Serves 4

Nonstick cooking spray
1 tablespoon low-sodium tamari or gluten-free soy sauce
Juice of 1 lemon
1 tablespoon honey
1 (1-inch) piece fresh ginger, grated
1 garlic clove, minced
1 pound (454 g) salmon fillet
¼ teaspoon salt, divided
⅛ teaspoon freshly ground black pepper
2 broccoli heads, cut into florets
1 tablespoon extra-virgin olive oil

Preheat the oven to 400°F (205°C). Spray a baking sheet with nonstick cooking spray. 2. In a small bowl, mix the tamari, lemon juice, honey, ginger, and garlic. Set aside. 3. Place the salmon skin-side down on the prepared baking sheet. Season with ⅛ teaspoon of salt and the pepper. 4. In a large mixing bowl, toss the broccoli and olive oil. Season with the remaining ⅛ teaspoon of salt. Arrange in a single layer on the baking sheet next to the salmon. Bake for 15 to 20 minutes until the salmon flakes easily with a fork and the broccoli is fork-tender. 5. In a small pan over medium heat, bring the tamari-ginger mixture to a simmer and cook for 1 to 2 minutes until it just begins to thicken. 6. Drizzle the sauce over the salmon and serve.

Per Serving

calories: 238 | fat: 11g | protein: 25g | carbs: 11g | sugars: 6g | fiber: 2g | sodium: 334mg

Lemon Pepper Salmon

Prep time: 5 minutes | Cook time: 20 minutes | Serves 4

Nonstick cooking spray	½ teaspoon freshly ground black pepper
¼ teaspoon salt	Zest and juice of ½ lemon
¼ teaspoon dried thyme	1 pound (454 g) salmon fillet

Preheat the oven to 425°F (220°C). Spray a baking sheet with nonstick cooking spray. 2. In a small bowl, combine the pepper, salt, lemon zest and juice, and thyme. Stir to combine. 3. Place the salmon on the prepared baking sheet, skin-side down. Spread the seasoning mixture evenly over the fillet. 4. Bake for 15 to 20 minutes, depending on the thickness of the fillet, until the flesh flakes easily.

Per Serving

calories: 163 | fat: 7g | protein: 23g | carbs: 1g | sugars: 0g | fiber: 0g | sodium: 167mg

Salsa Verde Baked Salmon

Prep time: 5 minutes | Cook time: 25 minutes | Serves 4

Nonstick cooking spray	8 ounces (227 g) tomatillos, husks removed
½ onion, quartered	1 jalapeño or serrano pepper, seeded
1 garlic clove, unpeeled	1 teaspoon extra-virgin olive oil
½ teaspoon salt, divided	4 (4-ounce / 113-g) wild-caught salmon fillets
¼ teaspoon freshly ground black pepper	¼ cup chopped fresh cilantro
Juice of 1 lime	

Preheat the oven to 425°F (220°C). Spray a baking sheet with nonstick cooking spray. 2. In a large bowl, toss the tomatillos, onion, jalapeño, garlic, olive oil, and ¼ teaspoon of salt to coat. Arrange in a single layer on the prepared baking sheet, and roast for about 10 minutes until just softened. Transfer to a dish or plate and set aside. 3. Arrange the salmon fillets skin-side down on the same baking sheet, and season with the remaining ¼ teaspoon of salt and the pepper. Bake for 12 to 15 minutes until the fish is firm and flakes easily. 4. Meanwhile, peel the roasted garlic and place it and the roasted vegetables in a blender or food processor. Add a scant ¼ cup of water to the jar, and process until smooth. 5. Add the cilantro and lime juice and process until smooth. Serve the salmon topped with the salsa verde.

Per Serving

calories: 199 | fat: 9g | protein: 23g | carbs: 6g | sugars: 3g | fiber: 2g | sodium: 295mg

Ceviche

Prep time: 10 minutes | Cook time: 0 minutes | Serves 4

½ pound (227 g) fresh skinless, white, ocean fish fillet (halibut, mahi mahi, etc.), diced	1 cup freshly squeezed lime juice, divided
	2 tablespoons chopped fresh cilantro, divided
1 serrano pepper, sliced	1 garlic clove, crushed
¾ teaspoon salt, divided	½ red onion, thinly sliced
2 tomatoes, diced	1 red bell pepper, seeded and diced
1 tablespoon extra-virgin olive oil	

In a large mixing bowl, combine the fish, ¾ cup of lime juice, 1 tablespoon of cilantro, serrano pepper, garlic, and ½ teaspoon of salt. The fish should be covered or nearly covered in lime juice. Cover the bowl and refrigerate for 4 hours. 2. Sprinkle the remaining ¼ teaspoon of salt over the onion in a small bowl, and let sit for 10 minutes. Drain and rinse well. 3. In a large bowl, combine the tomatoes, bell pepper, olive oil, remaining ¼ cup of lime juice, and onion. Let rest for at least 10 minutes, or as long as 4 hours, while the fish "cooks." 4. When the fish is ready, it will be completely white and opaque. At this time, strain the juice, reserving it in another bowl. If desired, remove the serrano pepper and garlic. 5. Add the vegetables to the fish, and stir gently. Taste, and add some of the reserved lime juice to the ceviche as desired. Serve topped with the remaining 1 tablespoon of cilantro.

Per Serving

calories: 121 | fat: 4g | protein: 12g | carbs: 11g | sugars: 5g | fiber: 2g | sodium: 405mg

Whole Veggie-Stuffed Trout

Prep time: 10 minutes | Cook time: 25 minutes | Serves 2

Nonstick cooking spray
(cleaned but with bones and skin intact)
¼ teaspoon salt
½ red bell pepper, seeded and thinly sliced
2 or 3 shiitake mushrooms, sliced
1 lemon, sliced

2 (8-ounce / 227-g) whole trout fillets, dressed
1 tablespoon extra-virgin olive oil
⅛ teaspoon freshly ground black pepper
1 small onion, thinly sliced
1 poblano pepper, seeded and thinly sliced

Preheat the oven to 425°F (220°C). Spray a baking sheet with nonstick cooking spray. 2. Rub both trout, inside and out, with the olive oil, then season with the salt and pepper. 3. In a large bowl, combine the bell pepper, onion, mushrooms, and poblano pepper. Stuff half of this mixture into the cavity of each fish. Top the mixture with 2 or 3 lemon slices inside each fish. 4. Arrange the fish on the prepared baking sheet side by side and roast for 25 minutes until the fish is cooked through and the vegetables are tender.

Per Serving

calories: 452 | fat: 22g | protein: 49g | carbs: 14g | sugars: 2g | fiber: 3g | sodium: 357mg

Honey Mustard Roasted Salmon

Prep time: 5 minutes | Cook time: 20 minutes | Serves 4

Nonstick cooking spray
1 tablespoon honey
¼ teaspoon salt
1 pound (454 g) salmon fillet

2 tablespoons whole-grain mustard
2 garlic cloves, minced
¼ teaspoon freshly ground black pepper

Preheat the oven to 425°F (220°C). Spray a baking sheet with nonstick cooking spray. 2. In a small bowl, whisk together the mustard, honey, garlic, salt, and pepper. Place the salmon fillet on the prepared baking sheet, skin-side down. Spoon the sauce onto the salmon and spread evenly. 3. Roast for 15 to 20 minutes, depending on the thickness of the fillet, until the flesh flakes easily.

Per Serving

calories: 186 | fat: 7g | protein: 23g | carbs: 6g | sugars: 4g | fiber: 0g | sodium: 312mg

Ginger-Garlic Fish in Parchment

Prep time: 10 minutes | Cook time: 15 minutes | Serves 4

1 chard bunch, stemmed, leaves and stems cut into thin strips
1 pound (454 g) cod fillets cut into 4 pieces
3 garlic cloves, minced
2 tablespoons low-sodium tamari or gluten-free soy sauce
1 red bell pepper, seeded and cut into strips
1 red bell pepper, seeded and cut into strips
1 tablespoon grated fresh ginger
2 tablespoons white wine vinegar
1 tablespoon honey

Preheat the oven to 425°F (220°C). 2. Cut four pieces of parchment paper, each about 16 inches wide. Lay the four pieces out on a large workspace. 3. On each piece of paper, arrange a small pile of chard leaves and stems, topped by several strips of bell pepper. Top with a piece of cod. 4. In a small bowl, mix the ginger, garlic, vinegar, tamari, and honey. Top each piece of fish with one-fourth of the mixture. 5. Fold the parchment paper over so the edges overlap. Fold the edges over several times to secure the fish in the packets. Carefully place the packets on a large baking sheet.
Bake for 12 minutes. Carefully open the packets, allowing steam to escape, and serve.

Per Serving

calories: 118 | fat: 1g | protein: 19g | carbs: 9g | sugars: 6g | fiber: 1g | sodium: 715mg

Blackened Tilapia with Mango Salsa

Prep time: 15 minutes | Cook time: 10 minutes | Serves 2

Salsa:
1 cup chopped mango
2 tablespoons chopped fresh cilantro
½ jalapeño pepper, seeded and minced
Tilapia:
1 tablespoon paprika
½ teaspoon freshly ground black pepper
½ teaspoon garlic powder
¼ teaspoon salt
2 teaspoons extra-virgin olive oil
2 tablespoons chopped red onion
2 tablespoons freshly squeezed lime juice
Pinch salt
1 teaspoon onion powder
½ teaspoon dried thyme
¼ teaspoon cayenne pepper
½ pound (227 g) boneless tilapia fillets
1 lime, cut into wedges, for serving

Make the Salsa
In a medium bowl, toss together the mango, onion, cilantro, lime juice, jalapeño, and salt. Set aside.
Make the Tilapia
In a small bowl, mix the paprika, onion powder, pepper, thyme, garlic powder, cayenne, and salt. Rub the mixture on both sides of the tilapia fillets. 2. In a large skillet, heat the oil over medium heat, and cook the fish for 3 to 5 minutes on each side until the outer coating is crisp and the fish is cooked through. 3. Spoon half of the salsa over each fillet and serve with lime wedges on the side.

Per Serving

calories: 240 | fat: 8g | protein: 25g | carbs: 22g | sugars: 13g | fiber: 4g | sodium: 417mg

Halibut Roasted with Green Beans

Prep time: 10 minutes | Cook time: 15 minutes | Serves 4

1 pound (454 g) green beans, trimmed
1 onion, sliced
3 garlic cloves, minced
1 teaspoon dried dill
4 (4-ounce / 113-g) halibut fillets
¼ teaspoon freshly ground black pepper

2 red bell peppers, seeded and cut into strips
Zest and juice of 2 lemons
2 tablespoons extra-virgin olive oil
1 teaspoon dried oregano
½ teaspoon salt

Preheat the oven to 400°F (205°C). Line a baking sheet with parchment paper. 2. In a large bowl, toss the green beans, bell peppers, onion, lemon zest and juice, garlic, olive oil, dill, and oregano. 3. Use a slotted spoon to transfer the vegetables to the prepared baking sheet in a single layer, leaving the juice behind in the bowl. 4. Gently place the halibut fillets in the bowl, and coat in the juice. Transfer the fillets to the baking sheet, nestled between the vegetables, and drizzle them with any juice left in the bowl. Sprinkle the vegetables and halibut with the salt and pepper. 5. Bake for 15 to 20 minutes until the vegetables are just tender and the fish flakes apart easily.

Per Serving

calories: 234 | fat: 9g | protein: 24g | carbs: 16g | sugars: 8g | fiber: 5g | sodium: 349mg

Seared Scallops with Asparagus

Prep time: 10 minutes | Cook time: 15 minutes | Serves 4

3 teaspoons extra-virgin olive oil, divided
1 pound (454 g) asparagus, trimmed and cut into 2-inch segments
1 tablespoon butter
1 pound (454 g) sea scallops
¼ cup dry white wine
Juice of 1 lemon
2 garlic cloves, minced
¼ teaspoon freshly ground black pepper

In a large skillet, heat 1½ teaspoons of oil over medium heat. 2. Add the asparagus and sauté for 5 to 6 minutes until just tender, stirring regularly. Remove from the skillet and cover with aluminum foil to keep warm. 3. Add the remaining 1½ teaspoons of oil and the butter to the skillet. When the butter is melted and sizzling, place the scallops in a single layer in the skillet. Cook for about 3 minutes on one side until nicely browned. Use tongs to gently loosen and flip the scallops, and cook on the other side for another 3 minutes until browned and cooked through. Remove and cover with foil to keep warm. 4. In the same skillet, combine the wine, lemon juice, garlic, and pepper. Bring to a simmer for 1 to 2 minutes, stirring to mix in any browned pieces left in the pan. 5. Return the asparagus and the cooked scallops to the skillet to coat with the sauce. Serve warm.

Per Serving

calories: 252 | fat: 7g | protein: 26g | carbs: 15g | sugars: 3g | fiber: 2g | sodium: 493mg

Baked Oysters with Vegetables

Prep time: 30 minutes | Cook time: 15 minutes | Serves 2

2 cups coarse salt, for holding the oysters
1 tablespoon butter
¼ cup finely chopped scallions, both white and green parts
1 garlic clove, minced
Zest and juice of ½ lemon
Freshly ground black pepper, to taste

1 dozen fresh oysters, scrubbed
½ cup finely chopped artichoke hearts
¼ cup finely chopped red bell pepper
¼ cup finely chopped red bell pepper
1 tablespoon finely chopped fresh parsley
Pinch salt

Pour the coarse salt into an 8-by-8-inch baking dish and spread to evenly fill the bottom of the dish. 2. Prepare a clean surface to shuck the oysters. Using a shucking knife, insert the blade at the joint of the shell, where it hinges open and shut. Firmly apply pressure to pop the blade in, and work the knife around the shell to open. Discard the empty half of the shell. Use the knife to gently loosen the oyster, and remove any shell particles. Set the oysters in their shells on the salt, being careful not to spill the juices. 3. Preheat the oven to 425ºF (220ºC). 4. In a large skillet, melt the butter over medium heat. Add the artichoke hearts, scallions, and bell pepper, and cook for 5 to 7 minutes. Add the garlic and cook an additional minute. Remove from the heat and mix in the parsley, lemon zest and juice, and season with salt and pepper. 5. Divide the vegetable mixture evenly among the oysters and bake for 10 to 12 minutes until the vegetables are lightly browned.

Per Serving
calories: 134 | fat: 7g | protein: 6g | carbs: 11g | sugars: 7g | fiber: 2g | sodium: 281mg

Cajun Shrimp and Quinoa Casserole

Prep time: 15 minutes | Cook time: 30 minutes | Serves 6

½ cup quinoa
1 pound (454 g) shrimp, peeled and deveined
4 tomatoes, diced
½ onion, diced
3 garlic cloves, minced
¼ teaspoon freshly ground black pepper

1 cup water
1½ teaspoons Cajun seasoning, divided
1 tablespoon plus 2 teaspoons extra-virgin olive oil, divided
1 jalapeño pepper, seeded and minced
1 tablespoon tomato paste
½ cup shredded pepper jack cheese

In a pot, combine the quinoa and water. Bring to a boil, reduce the heat, cover, and simmer on low for 10 to 15 minutes until all the water is absorbed. Fluff with a fork. 2. Preheat the oven to 350ºF (180ºC). 3. In a large mixing bowl, toss the shrimp and ¾ teaspoon of Cajun seasoning. 4. In another bowl, toss the remaining ¾ teaspoon of Cajun seasoning with the tomatoes and 1½ teaspoons of olive oil. 5. In a large, oven-safe skillet, heat 1 tablespoon of olive oil over medium heat. Add the shrimp and cook for 2 to 3 minutes per side until they are opaque and firm. Remove from the skillet and set aside. 6. In the same skillet, heat the remaining ½ teaspoon of olive oil over medium-high heat. Add the onion, jalapeño, and garlic, and cook until the onion softens, 3 to 5 minutes. 7. Add the seasoned tomatoes, tomato paste, cooked quinoa, and pepper. Stir well to combine. 8. Return the shrimp to the skillet, placing them in a single layer on top of the quinoa. Sprinkle the cheese over the top. Transfer the skillet to the oven and bake for 15 minutes. Turn the broiler on high, and broil for 2 minutes to brown the cheese. Serve.

Per Serving
calories: 255 | fat: 12g | protein: 18g | carbs: 15g | sugars: 1g | fiber: 2g | sodium: 469mg

Shrimp Burgers with Mango Salsa

Prep time: 15 minutes | Cook time: 10 minutes | Serves 4

Salsa:

1 cup diced mango

1 scallion, both white and green parts, finely chopped

Juice of 1 lime

1 avocado, diced

1 tablespoon chopped fresh cilantro

1 tablespoon chopped fresh cilantro

¼ teaspoon freshly ground black pepper

Burgers:

1 pound (454 g) shrimp, peeled and deveined

½ red bell pepper, seeded and coarsely chopped

2 tablespoons fresh chopped cilantro

¼ teaspoon freshly ground black pepper

4 cups mixed salad greens

1 large egg

¼ cup chopped scallions, both white and green parts

2 garlic cloves

1 tablespoon extra-virgin olive oil

Make the Salsa

1.In a small bowl, toss the mango, avocado, scallion, and cilantro. Sprinkle with the lime juice and pepper. Mix gently to combine and set aside.

Make the Burgers

In the bowl of a food processor, add half the shrimp and process until coarsely puréed. Add the egg, bell pepper, scallions, cilantro, and garlic, and process until uniformly chopped. Transfer to a large mixing bowl. 2. Using a sharp knife, chop the remaining half pound of shrimp into small pieces. Add to the puréed mixture and stir well to combine. Add the pepper and stir well. Form the mixture into 4 patties of equal size. Arrange on a plate, cover, and refrigerate for 30 minutes. 3. In a large skillet, heat the olive oil over medium heat. Cook the burgers for 3 minutes on each side until browned and cooked through. 4. On each of 4 plates, arrange 1 cup of salad greens, and top with a scoop of salsa and a shrimp burger.

Per Serving

calories: 229 | fat: 11g | protein: 19g | carbs: 14g | sugars: 7g | fiber: 4g | sodium: 200mg

Open-Faced Tuna Melts

Prep time: 5 minutes | Cook time: 5 minutes | Serves 3

3 English muffins, 100% whole-wheat

2 (5-ounce / 142-g) cans chunk-light tuna, drained

3 tablespoons plain low-fat Greek yogurt

½ teaspoon freshly ground black pepper

¾ cup shredded Cheddar cheese

If your broiler is in the top of your oven, place the oven rack in the center position. Turn the broiler on high. 2. Split the English muffins, if necessary, and toast them in the toaster. 3. Meanwhile, in a medium bowl, mix the tuna, yogurt, and pepper. 4. Place the muffin halves on a baking sheet, and spoon one-sixth of the tuna mixture and 2 tablespoons of Cheddar cheese on top of each half. Broil for 2 minutes or until the cheese melts.

Per Serving

calories: 392 | fat: 13g | protein: 40g | carbs: 28g | sugars: 6g | fiber: 5g | sodium: 474mg

Shrimp Stir-Fry

Prep time: 5 minutes | Cook time: 15 minutes | Serves 4

Sauce:

½ cup water

2 tablespoons honey

¼ teaspoon garlic powder

1 tablespoon cornstarch

2½ tablespoons low-sodium soy sauce

1 tablespoon rice vinegar

Pinch ground ginger

Stir-Fry:

8 cups frozen vegetable stir-fry mix

40 medium fresh shrimp, peeled and deveined

2 tablespoons sesame oil

Make the Sauce

In a small saucepan, whisk together the water, soy sauce, honey, rice vinegar, garlic powder, and ginger. Add the cornstarch and whisk until fully incorporated. 2. Bring the sauce to a boil over medium heat. Boil for 1 minute to thicken. Remove the sauce from the heat and set aside.

Make the Stir-Fry

Heat a large saucepan over medium-high heat. When hot, put the vegetable stir-fry mix into the pan, and cook for 7 to 10 minutes, stirring occasionally until the water completely evaporates. 2. Reduce the heat to medium-low, add the oil and shrimp, and stir. Cook for about 3 minutes, or until the shrimp are pink and opaque.

Add the sauce to the shrimp and vegetables and stir to coat. Cook for 2 minutes more.

Per Serving

calories: 297 | fat: 17g | protein: 24g | carbs: 14g | sugars: 9g | fiber: 2g | sodium: 454mg

Fish Tacos

Prep time: 5 minutes | Cook time: 10 minutes | Serves 4

Tacos:

2 tablespoons extra-virgin olive oil

8 (10-inch) yellow corn tortillas

¼ cup chopped fresh cilantro

4 (6-ounce / 170-g) cod fillets

2 cups packaged shredded cabbage

4 lime wedges

Sauce:

½ cup plain low-fat Greek yogurt

½ teaspoon garlic powder

⅓ cup low-fat mayonnaise

½ teaspoon ground cumin

Make the Tacos

Heat a medium skillet over medium-low heat. When hot, pour the oil into the skillet, then add the fish and cover. Cook for 4 minutes, then flip and cook for 4 minutes more. 2. Top each tortilla with one-eighth of the cabbage, sauce, cilantro, and fish. Finish each taco with a squeeze of lime.

Make the Sauce

In a small bowl, whisk together the yogurt, mayonnaise, garlic powder, and cumin.

Per Serving

calories: 373 | fat: 13g | protein: 36g | carbs: 30g | sugars: 4g | fiber: 4g | sodium: 342mg

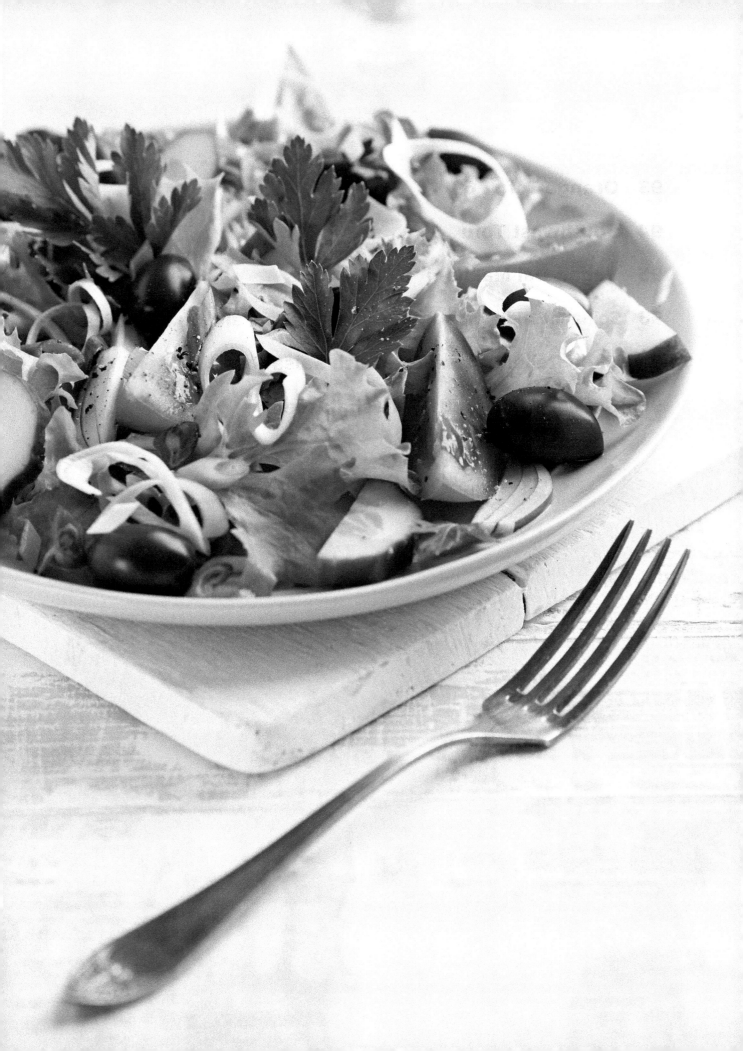

Chapter 7 Vegetarian Mains

Orange Tofu

Prep time: 10 minutes | Cook time: 20 minutes | Serves 4

⅓ cup freshly squeezed orange juice (zest orange first; see orange zest ingredient below)
1 tablespoon tamari
1 tablespoon tahini
½ tablespoon coconut nectar or pure maple syrup
2 tablespoons apple cider vinegar
½ tablespoon freshly grated ginger
1 large clove garlic, grated
½-1 teaspoon orange zest
¼ teaspoon sea salt
Few pinches of crushed red-pepper flakes (optional)
1 package (12 ounces) extra-firm tofu, sliced into ¼"-½» thick squares and patted to remove excess moisture

1. Preheat the oven to 400°F. 2. In a small bowl, combine the orange juice, tamari, tahini, nectar or syrup, vinegar, ginger, garlic, orange zest, salt, and red-pepper flakes (if using). Whisk until well combined. Pour the sauce into an 8" × 12" baking dish. Add the tofu and turn to coat both sides. Bake for 20 minutes. Add salt to taste.

Per Serving
Calorie: 122 | fat: 7g | protein: 10g | carbs: 7g | sugars: 4g | fiber: 1g | sodium: 410mg

Southwest Tofu

Prep time: 10 minutes | Cook time: 20 minutes | Serves 4

3½ tablespoons freshly squeezed lime juice
2 teaspoons pure maple syrup
1½ teaspoons ground cumin
1 teaspoon dried oregano leaves
1 teaspoon chili powder
½ teaspoon paprika
½ teaspoon sea salt
⅛ teaspoon allspice
1 package (12 ounces) extra-firm tofu, sliced into ¼"-½» thick squares and patted to remove excess moisture

1. In a 9" × 12" baking dish, combine the lime juice, syrup, cumin, oregano, chili powder, paprika, salt, and allspice. Add the tofu and turn to coat both sides. Bake uncovered for 20 minutes, or until the marinade is absorbed, turning once.

Per Serving
Calorie: 78 | fat: 4g | protein: 7g | carbs: 6g | sugars: 3g | fiber: 1g | sodium: 324mg

Vegan Dal Makhani

Prep time: 0 minutes | Cook time: 55 minutes | Serves 6

1 cup dried kidney beans

⅓ cup urad dal or beluga or Puy lentils

4 cups water

1 teaspoon fine sea salt

1 tablespoon cold-pressed avocado oil

1 tablespoon cumin seeds

1-inch piece fresh ginger, peeled and minced

4 garlic cloves, minced

1 large yellow onion, diced

2 jalapeño chiles, seeded and diced

1 green bell pepper, seeded and diced

1 tablespoon garam masala

1 teaspoon ground turmeric

¼ teaspoon cayenne pepper (optional)

1(15-ounce / 425-g / 425-g) can fire-roasted diced tomatoes and liquid

2 tablespoons vegan buttery spread

Cooked cauliflower "rice" for serving

2 tablespoons chopped fresh cilantro

6 tablespoons plain coconut yogurt

1. In a medium bowl, combine the kidney beans, urad dal, water, and salt and stir to dissolve the salt. Let soak for 12 hours. 2. Select the Sauté setting on the Instant Pot and heat the oil and cumin seeds for 3 minutes, until the seeds are bubbling, lightly toasted, and aromatic. Add the ginger and garlic and sauté for 1 minute, until bubbling and fragrant. Add the onion, jalapeños, and bell pepper and sauté for 5 minutes, until the onion begins to soften. 3. Add the garam masala, turmeric, cayenne (if using), and the soaked beans and their liquid and stir to mix. Pour the tomatoes and their liquid on top. Do not stir them in. 4. Secure the lid and set the Pressure Release to Sealing. Press the Cancel button to reset the cooking program, then select the Pressure Cook or Manual setting and set the cooking time for 30 minutes at high pressure. (The pot will take about 15 minutes to come up to pressure before the cooking program begins.) 5. When the cooking program ends, let the pressure release naturally for 30 minutes, then move the Pressure Release to Venting to release any remaining steam. Open the pot and stir to combine, then stir in the buttery spread. If you prefer a smoother texture, ladle 1½ cups of the dal into a blender and blend until smooth, about 30 seconds, then stir the blended mixture into the rest of the dal in the pot. 6. Spoon the cauliflower "rice" into bowls and ladle the dal on top. Sprinkle with the cilantro, top with a dollop of coconut yogurt, and serve.

Per Serving

Calorie: 245 | fat: 7g | protein: 11g | carbs: 37g | sugars: 4g | fiber: 10g | sodium: 518mg

Spinach Salad with Eggs, Tempeh Bacon, and Strawberries

Prep time: 10 minutes | Cook time: 15 minutes | Serves 4

2 tablespoons soy sauce, tamari, or coconut aminos

1 tablespoon raw apple cider vinegar

1 tablespoon pure maple syrup

½ teaspoon smoked paprika

Freshly ground black pepper

1 (8-ounce / 227-g) package tempeh, cut crosswise into ⅛-inch-thick slices

8 large eggs

3 tablespoons extra-virgin olive oil

1 shallot, minced

1 tablespoon red wine vinegar

1 tablespoon balsamic vinegar

1 teaspoon Dijon mustard

¼ teaspoon fine sea salt

1 (6-ounce /170-g) bag baby spinach

2 hearts romaine lettuce, torn into bite-size pieces

12 fresh strawberries, sliced

1. In a 1-quart ziplock plastic bag, combine the soy sauce, cider vinegar, maple syrup, paprika, and ½ teaspoon pepper and carefully agitate the bag to mix the ingredients to make a marinade. Add the tempeh, seal the bag, and turn the bag back and forth several times to coat the tempeh evenly with the marinade. Marinate in the refrigerator for at least 2 hours or up to 24 hours. 2. Pour 1 cup water into the Instant Pot and place the wire metal steam rack, an egg rack, or a steamer basket into the pot. Gently place the eggs on top of the rack or in the basket, taking care not to crack them. 3. Secure the lid and set the Pressure Release to Sealing. Select the Steam setting and set the cooking time for 3 minutes at high pressure. (The pot will take about 5 minutes to come up to pressure before the cooking program begins.) 4. While the eggs are cooking, prepare an ice bath. 5. When the cooking program ends, perform a quick pressure release by moving the Pressure Release to Venting. Open the pot and, using tongs, transfer the eggs to the ice bath to cool. 6. Remove the tempeh from the marinade and blot dry between layers of paper towels. Discard the marinade. In a large nonstick skillet over medium-high heat, warm 1 tablespoon of the oil for 2 minutes. Add the tempeh in a single layer and fry, turning once, for 2 to 3 minutes per side, until well browned. Transfer the tempeh to a plate and set aside. 7. Wipe out the skillet and set it over medium heat. Add the remaining 2 tablespoons oil and the shallot and sauté for about 2 minutes, until the shallot is golden brown. Turn off the heat and stir in the red wine vinegar, balsamic vinegar, mustard, salt, and ¼ teaspoon pepper to make a vinaigrette. 8. In a large bowl, combine the spinach and romaine. Pour in the vinaigrette and toss until all of the leaves are lightly coated. Divide the dressed greens evenly among four large serving plates or shallow bowls and arrange the strawberries and fried tempeh on top. Peel the eggs, cut them in half lengthwise, and place them on top of the salads. Top with a couple grinds of pepper and serve right away.

Per Serving

Calorie: 435 | fat: 25g | protein: 29g | carbs: 25g | sugars: 10g | fiber: 5g | sodium: 332mg

Chile Relleno Casserole with Salsa Salad

Prep time: 10 minutes | Cook time: 55 minutes | Serves 4

Casserole

½ cup gluten-free flour (such as King Arthur or Cup4Cup brand)

1 teaspoon baking powder

6 large eggs

½ cup nondairy milk or whole milk

3 (4-ounce / 113-g) cans fire-roasted diced green chiles, drained

1 cup nondairy cheese shreds or shredded mozzarella cheese

Salad

1 head green leaf lettuce, shredded

2 Roma tomatoes, seeded and diced

1 green bell pepper, seeded and diced

½ small yellow onion, diced

1 jalapeño chile, seeded and diced (optional)

2 tablespoons chopped fresh cilantro

4 teaspoons extra-virgin olive oil

4 teaspoons fresh lime juice

⅛ teaspoon fine sea salt

1. To make the casserole: Pour 1 cup water into the Instant Pot. Butter a 7-cup round heatproof glass dish or coat with nonstick cooking spray and place the dish on a long-handled silicone steam rack. (If you don't have the long-handled rack, use the wire metal steam rack and a homemade sling) 2. In a medium bowl, whisk together the flour and baking powder. Add the eggs and milk and whisk until well blended, forming a batter. Stir in the chiles and ¾ cup of the cheese. 3. Pour the batter into the prepared dish and cover tightly with aluminum foil. Holding the handles of the steam rack, lower the dish into the Instant Pot. 4. Secure the lid and set the Pressure Release to Sealing. Select the Pressure Cook or Manual setting and set the cooking time for 40 minutes at high pressure. (The pot will take about 10 minutes to come up to pressure before the cooking program begins.) 5. When the cooking program ends, let the pressure release naturally for at least 10 minutes, then move the Pressure Release to Venting to release any remaining steam. Open the pot and, wearing heat-resistant mitts, grasp the handles of the steam rack and lift it out of the pot. Uncover the dish, taking care not to get burned by the steam or to drip condensation onto the casserole. While the casserole is still piping hot, sprinkle the remaining ¼ cup cheese evenly on top. Let the cheese melt for 5 minutes. 6. To make the salad: While the cheese is melting, in a large bowl, combine the lettuce, tomatoes, bell pepper, onion, jalapeño (if using), cilantro, oil, lime juice, and salt. Toss until evenly combined. 7. Cut the casserole into wedges. Serve warm, with the salad on the side.

Per Serving

Calorie: 361 | fat: 22g | protein: 21g | carbs: 23g | sugars: 8g | fiber: 3g | sodium: 421mg

No-Bake Spaghetti Squash Casserole

Prep time: 10 minutes | Cook time: 45 minutes | Serves 6

Marinara

3 tablespoons extra-virgin olive oil
1 (28-ounce / 794-g) can whole San Marzano tomatoes and their liquid
1 teaspoon fine sea salt

3 garlic cloves, minced
2 teaspoons Italian seasoning
2 teaspoons Italian seasoning
½ teaspoon red pepper flakes (optional)

Vegan Parmesan

½ cup raw whole cashews
½ teaspoon garlic powder

2 tablespoons nutritional yeast
½ teaspoon fine sea salt

Vegan Ricotta

1 (14-ounce / 397-g) package firm tofu, drained
½ cup raw whole cashews, soaked in water to cover for 1 to 2 hours and then drained
3 tablespoons nutritional yeast
2 tablespoons extra-virgin olive oil
1 teaspoon finely grated lemon zest, plus 2 tablespoons fresh lemon juice
½ cup firmly packed fresh flat-leaf parsley leaves
1½ teaspoons Italian seasoning
1 teaspoon garlic powder
1 teaspoon fine sea salt
½ teaspoon freshly ground black pepper
One 3½-pound steamed spaghetti squash
2 tablespoons chopped fresh flat-leaf parsley

1. To make the marinara: Select the Sauté setting on the Instant Pot and heat the oil and garlic for about 2 minutes, until the garlic is bubbling but not browned. Add the tomatoes and their liquid and use a wooden spoon or spatula to crush the tomatoes against the side of the pot. Stir in the Italian seasoning, salt, and pepper flakes (if using) and cook, stirring occasionally, for about 10 minutes, until the sauce has thickened a bit. Press the Cancel button to turn off the pot and let the sauce cook from the residual heat for about 5 minutes more, until it is no longer simmering. Wearing heat-resistant mitts, lift the pot out of the housing, pour the sauce into a medium heatproof bowl, and set aside. (You can make the sauce up to 4 days in advance, then let it cool, transfer it to an airtight container, and refrigerate.) 2. To make the vegan Parmesan: In a food processor, combine the cashews, nutritional yeast, garlic powder, and salt. Using 1-second pulses, pulse about ten times, until the mixture resembles grated Parmesan cheese. Transfer to a small bowl and set aside. Do not wash the food processor bowl and blade. 3. To make the vegan ricotta: Cut the tofu crosswise into eight ½-inch-thick slices. Sandwich the slices between double layers of paper towels or a folded kitchen towel and press gently to remove excess moisture. Add the tofu to the food processor along with the cashews, nutritional yeast, oil, lemon zest, lemon juice, parsley, Italian seasoning, garlic powder, salt, and pepper. Process for about 1 minute, until the mixture is mostly smooth with flecks of parsley throughout. Set aside. 4. Return the marinara to the pot. Select the Sauté setting and heat the marinara sauce for about 3 minutes, until it starts to simmer. Add the spaghetti squash and vegan ricotta to the pot and stir to combine. Continue to heat, stirring often, for 8 to 10 minutes, until piping hot. Press the Cancel button to turn off the pot. 5. Spoon the spaghetti squash into bowls, top with the vegan Parmesan and parsley, and serve right away.

Per Serving

Calorie: 307 | fat: 17g | protein: 16g | carbs: 25g | sugars: 2g | fiber: 5g | sodium: 985mg

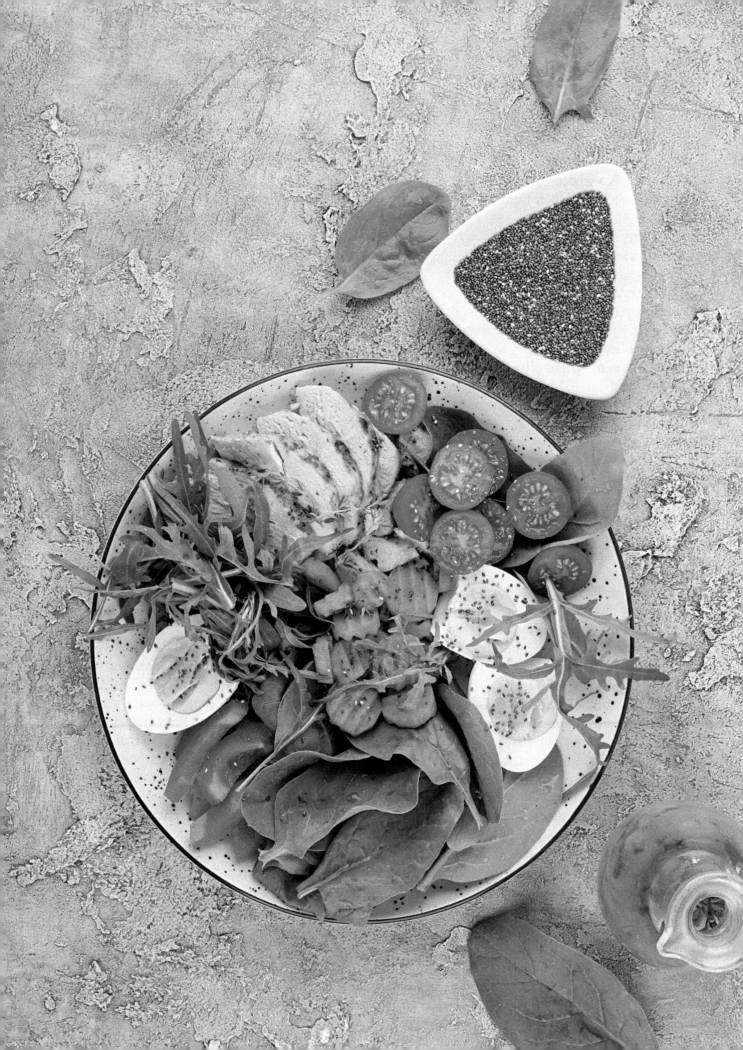

Chapter 8 Snacks and Appetizers

Greek Salad Kabobs

Prep time: 15 minutes | Cook time: 0 minutes | Serves 24

Dip
¾ cup plain fat-free yogurt

2 teaspoons chopped fresh dill weed

¼ teaspoon salt

2 teaspoons honey

2 teaspoons chopped fresh oregano leaves

1 small clove garlic, finely chopped

Kabobs
24 cocktail picks or toothpicks

24 small grape tomatoes

12 slices (½ inch) English (seedless) cucumber, cut in half crosswise

24 pitted kalamata olives

1. In small bowl, mix dip ingredients; set aside. 2. On each cocktail pick, thread 1 olive, 1 tomato and 1 half-slice cucumber. Serve kabobs with dip.

Per Serving
Calorie: 15 | fat: 0g | protein: 0g | carbs: 2g | sugars: 1g | fiber: 0g | sodium: 70mg

Green Goddess White Bean Dip

Prep time: 1 minutes | Cook time: 45 minutes | Makes 3 cups

1 cup dried navy, great Northern, or cannellini beans

2 teaspoons fine sea salt

¼ cup extra-virgin olive oil, plus 1 tablespoon

1 bunch chives, chopped

Freshly ground black pepper

4 cups water

4 cups water

3 tablespoons fresh lemon juice

¼ cup firmly packed fresh flat-leaf parsley leaves

Leaves from 2 tarragon sprigs

1. Combine the beans, water, and 1 teaspoon of the salt in the Instant Pot and stir to dissolve the salt. 2. Secure the lid and set the Pressure Release to Sealing. Select the Bean/Chili, Pressure Cook, or Manual setting and set the cooking time for 30 minutes at high pressure if using navy or Great Northern beans or 40 minutes at high pressure if using cannellini beans. (The pot will take about 15 minutes to come up to pressure before the cooking program begins.) 3. When the cooking program ends, let the pressure release naturally for 15 minutes, then move the Pressure Release to Venting to release any remaining steam. Open the pot and scoop out and reserve ½ cup of the cooking liquid. Wearing heat-resistant mitts, lift out the inner pot and drain the beans in a colander. 4. In a food processor or blender, combine the beans, ½ cup cooking liquid, lemon juice, ¼ cup olive oil, ½ teaspoon parsley, chives, tarragon, remaining 1 teaspoon salt, and ½ teaspoon pepper. Process or blend on medium speed, stopping to scrape down the sides of the container as needed, for about 1 minute, until the mixture is smooth. 5. Transfer the dip to a serving bowl. Drizzle with the remaining 1 tablespoon olive oil and sprinkle with a few grinds of pepper. The dip will keep in an airtight container in the refrigerator for up to 1 week. Serve at room temperature or chilled.

Per Serving
Calorie: 70 | fat: 5g | protein: 3g | carbs: 8g | sugars: 1g | fiber: 4g | sodium: 782mg

Lemon Cream Fruit Dip

Prep time: 5 minutes | Cook time: 0 minutes | Serves 4

1 cup (200 g) plain nonfat Greek yogurt
¼ cup (28 g) coconut flour 1 tablespoon (15 ml) pure maple syrup
½ teaspoon pure vanilla extract
½ teaspoon pure almond extract
Zest of 1 medium lemon
Juice of ½ medium lemon

1. In a medium bowl, whisk together the yogurt, coconut flour, maple syrup, vanilla, almond extract, lemon zest, and lemon juice. Serve the dip with fruit or crackers.

Per Serving

Calorie: 80 | fat: 1g | protein: 7g | carbs: 10g | sugars: 6g | fiber: 3g | sodium: 37mg

Vietnamese Meatball Lollipops with Dipping Sauce

Prep time: 30 minutes | Cook time: 20 minutes | Serves 12

Meatballs
1¼ pounds lean (at least 90%) ground turkey
¼ cup chopped water chestnuts, from (8-ounce /227-g) can, drained
¼ cup chopped fresh cilantro
1 tablespoon cornstarch
2 tablespoons fish sauce
½ teaspoon pepper
3 cloves garlic, finely chopped
Dipping Sauce
¼ cup water
¼ cup reduced-sodium soy sauce
2 tablespoons packed brown sugar
2 tablespoons chopped fresh chives or green onions
2 tablespoons lime juice
2 cloves garlic, finely chopped
½ teaspoon crushed red pepper
About 24 (6-inch) bamboo skewers

1. Heat oven to 400°F. Line cookie sheet with foil; spray with cooking spray (or use nonstick foil). 2. In large bowl, combine all meatball ingredients until well mixed. Shape into 1¼-inch meatballs. On cookie sheet, place meatballs 1 inch apart. Bake 20 minutes, turning halfway through baking, until thermometer inserted in center of meatballs reads at least 165°F. 3. Meanwhile, in 1-quart saucepan, heat all dipping sauce ingredients over low heat until sugar is dissolved; set aside. 4. Insert bamboo skewers into cooked meatballs; place on serving plate. Serve with warm dipping sauce.

Per Serving

Calorie: 80 | fat: 2g | protein: 10g | carbs: 5g | sugars: 3g | fiber: 0g | sodium: 440mg

Blackberry Baked Brie

Prep time: 5 minutes | Cook time: 15 minutes | Serves 5

8 ounces round Brie
1 cup water
¼ cup sugar-free blackberry preserves
2 teaspoons chopped fresh mint

1. Slice a grid pattern into the top of the rind of the Brie with a knife. 2. In a 7-inch round baking dish, place the Brie, then cover the baking dish securely with foil. 3. Insert the trivet into the inner pot of the Instant Pot; pour in the water. 4. Make a foil sling and arrange it on top of the trivet. Place the baking dish on top of the trivet and foil sling. 5. Secure the lid to the locked position and turn the vent to sealing. 6. Press Manual and set the Instant Pot for 15 minutes on high pressure. 7. When cooking time is up, turn off the Instant Pot and do a quick release of the pressure. 8. When the valve has dropped, remove the lid, then remove the baking dish. 9. Remove the top rind of the Brie and top with the preserves. Sprinkle with the fresh mint.

Per Serving
Calorie: 133 | fat: 10g | protein: 8g | carbs: 4g | sugars: 0g | fiber: 0g | sodium: 238mg

Creamy Spinach Dip

Prep time: 13 minutes | Cook time: 5 minutes | Serves 11

8 ounces low-fat cream cheese
1 cup low-fat sour cream
½ cup finely chopped onion
½ cup no-sodium vegetable broth
5 cloves garlic, minced
½ teaspoon salt
¼ teaspoon black pepper
10 ounces (283 g) frozen spinach
12 ounces reduced-fat shredded Monterey Jack cheese
12 ounces reduced-fat shredded Parmesan cheese

1. Add cream cheese, sour cream, onion, vegetable broth, garlic, salt, pepper, and spinach to the inner pot of the Instant Pot. 2. Secure lid, make sure vent is set to sealing, and set to the Bean/Chili setting on high pressure for 5 minutes. 3. When done, do a manual release. 4. Add the cheeses and mix well until creamy and well combined.

Per Serving
Calorie: 274 | fat: 18g | protein: 19g | carbs: 10g | sugars: 3g | fiber: 1g | sodium: 948mg

Chapter 9 Pasta

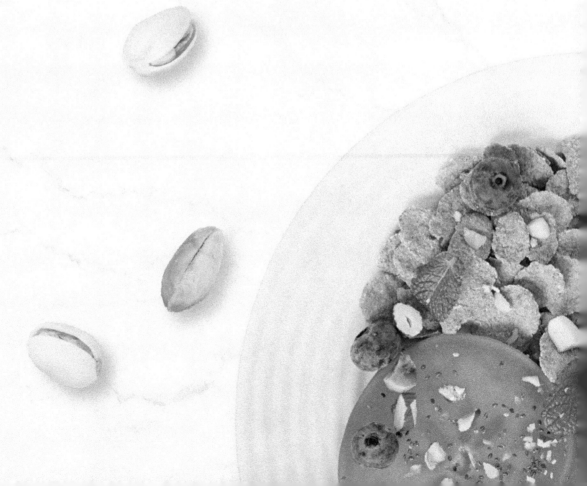

Whole Wheat Lasagna Wheels

Prep time: 30 minutes | Cook time: 40 minutes | Serves 4

8 uncooked whole wheat lasagna noodles
3 cups sliced cremini mushrooms
2 small zucchini, unpeeled, halved lengthwise and sliced
½ teaspoon pepper
1 cup part-skim ricotta cheese
½ cup shredded part-skim mozzarella cheese
¼ cup grated Parmesan cheese
½ cup chopped fresh basil leaves
1½ cups tomato pasta sauce

1 Heat oven to 350°F. Spray 13x9-inch (3-quart) glass baking dish with cooking spray. Cook noodles as directed on package. Drain; rinse with cold water to cool. Drain well; lay noodles flat. 2. Meanwhile, spray 10-inch skillet with cooking spray. Heat over medium-high heat. Add mushrooms and zucchini to skillet; sprinkle with pepper. Cook 5 to 8 minutes, stirring frequently, until vegetables are very tender. Remove from heat. Drain; return to skillet. Stir in ricotta cheese, mozzarella cheese, Parmesan cheese and basil until well blended. 3. In baking dish, spread ½ cup pasta sauce. For each lasagna wheel, spoon ⅓ cup vegetable mixture on center of each cooked noodle; spread to ends. Carefully roll up from short end, forming wheel. Place wheels, seam-side down, in baking dish. Spoon remaining 1 cup sauce evenly over tops of lasagna wheels. 4. Cover and bake 30 minutes or until sauce is bubbly. Serve warm, spooning sauce from baking dish over top of each lasagna wheel.

Per Serving
Calorie: 400 | fat: 11g | protein: 22g | carbs: 50g | sugars: 17g | fiber: 6g | sodium: 740mg

Pesto Pasta in a Pinch

Prep time: 10 minutes | Cook time: 0 minutes | Serves 4

½ cup (12 g) fresh basil leaves
½ cup (15 g) baby spinach
2 tablespoons (14 g) coarsely chopped walnuts
½ tablespoon (5 g) minced garlic
¼ cup (60 ml) olive oil
¼ cup (32 g) crumbled feta cheese
8 ounces (227 g) chickpea or lentil pasta, cooked
1 cup (149 g) halved grape tomatoes

1. In a food processor or blender, combine the basil, spinach, walnuts, garlic, oil, and feta cheese. Process the ingredients for 30 to 45 seconds, until they are homogeneous. 2. Place the pasta in a medium bowl. Pour the pesto over the pasta and toss to coat it in the sauce. 3. Gently fold in the tomatoes, then serve the pasta.

Per Serving
Calorie: 374 | fat: 21g | protein: 13g | carbs: 38g | sugars: 2g | fiber: 6g | sodium: 139mg

Slow Cooker Mediterranean Minestrone Casserole

Prep time: 20 minutes | Cook time: 6 to 8 hours | Serves 6

3 medium carrots, sliced (1½ cups)

1 cup water

1½ teaspoons dried Italian seasoning

1 can (28 ounces) diced tomatoes, undrained

drained, rinsed

2 cloves garlic, finely chopped

1 cup uncooked elbow macaroni

1 medium onion, chopped (½ cup)

2 teaspoons sugar

¼ teaspoon pepper

1 can (15 ounces) chickpeas (garbanzo beans),

1 can (6 ounces / 170-g) no-salt-added tomato paste

1½ cups frozen cut green beans, thawed

½ cup shredded Parmesan cheese (2 ounces)

1 In 3- to 4-quart slow cooker, mix all ingredients except green beans, macaroni and cheese. 2. Cover; cook on Low heat setting 6 to 8 hours. 3. About 20 minutes before serving, stir in green beans and macaroni. Increase heat setting to High. Cover; cook about 20 minutes or until beans and macaroni are tender. Sprinkle with cheese.

Per Serving

Calorie: 340 | fat: 5g | protein: 16g | carbs: 57g | sugars: 13g | fiber: 9g | sodium: 510mg

Chunky Garden Noodles

Prep time: 30 minutes | Cook time: 15 minutes | Serves 6

Sauce

2 tablespoons olive oil

1 green bell pepper, chopped

3 cloves garlic, chopped

½ cup pimiento-stuffed green olives, chopped

1 tablespoon chopped fresh oregano leaves

¼ teaspoon salt

1 medium onion, chopped (1 cup)

3 cups sliced cremini mushrooms

1 can (28 ounces) crushed tomatoes, undrained

⅓ cup chopped fresh basil leaves

½ teaspoon crushed red pepper flakes

Noodles

2 packages (8 ounces each) tofu shirataki noodles, spaghetti style drained

Topping

¼ cup grated Parmesan cheese

1. In 2-quart saucepan, heat oil over medium-high heat. Add onion and bell pepper to oil; cook about 5 minutes, stirring frequently, until onion is tender. Stir in mushrooms and garlic; cook about 5 minutes, stirring frequently, until mushrooms are tender and liquid evaporates. Add remaining sauce ingredients; reduce heat. Cover; simmer, stirring occasionally, while preparing noodles. 2. In 3-quart saucepan, heat 2 quarts water to boiling. Add noodles. Cook 2 to 3 minutes; drain. On heatproof plate lined with paper towels, place noodles (to prevent them from sticking together). Divide warm noodles evenly among 6 bowls. For each serving, top noodles with 1 cup sauce and sprinkle with 2 teaspoons Parmesan cheese.

Per Serving

Calorie: 170 | fat: 8g | protein: 6g | carbs: 18g | sugars: 9g | fiber: 5g | sodium: 760mg

Pasta Carbonara

Prep time: 10 minutes | Cook time: 10 minutes | Serves 4

2 cups steamed cauliflower florets
⅓ cup soaked and drained raw cashews
1½ tablespoons chickpea miso (or other mild-flavored miso)
1-2 large cloves garlic
½ teaspoon sea salt
½ teaspoon black salt
1½ cups plain low-fat nondairy milk
2 tablespoons lemon juice
Few pinches of freshly grated nutmeg and/or black pepper
1 pound (454 g) dry pasta
½-¾ cup frozen peas (optional)
¼-⅓ cup water

Boil the water for the pasta. Meanwhile, in a blender, combine the cauliflower, cashews, miso, garlic, sea salt, black salt, milk, lemon juice, and nutmeg and/or pepper. 2. Puree until very smooth. Prepare the pasta according to package directions. Once the pasta is almost cooked (still having some "bite," not mushy), add the peas to the cooking water and then immediately drain, and return the pasta and peas to the pot. Pour the sauce from the blender into the pot. 3. Use the water to swish and rinse any remaining sauce from the blender into the pot. Gently heat the pasta and sauce over medium-low heat for a minute or two, or until the sauce thickens. Taste, and add additional salt and pepper if

Per Serving
Calorie: 616 | fat: 9g | protein: 24g | carbs: 110g | sugars: 7g | fiber: 8g | sodium: 875mg

Chapter 10 Desserts

Frozen Mocha Milkshake

Prep time: 5 minutes | Cook time: 0 minutes | Serves 1

1 cup (240 ml) unsweetened vanilla almond milk
3 tablespoons (18 g) unsweetened cocoa powder
2 teaspoons (4 g) instant espresso powder
1½ cups (210 g) crushed ice
½ medium avocado, peeled and pitted
1 tablespoon (15 ml) pure maple syrup
1 teaspoon pure vanilla extract

1. In a blender, combine the almond milk, cocoa powder, espresso powder, ice, avocado, maple syrup, and vanilla. Blend the ingredients on high speed for 60 seconds, until the milkshake is smooth.

Per Serving
Calorie: 307 | fat: 20g | protein: 6g | carbs: 33g | sugars: 13g | fiber: 13g | sodium: 173mg

Baked Berry Cups with Crispy Cinnamon Wedges

Prep time: 25 minutes | Cook time: 30 minutes | Serves 4

2 teaspoons sugar
¾ teaspoon ground cinnamon
Butter-flavor cooking spray
1 balanced carb whole wheat tortilla (6 inch)
¼ cup sugar
2 tablespoons white whole wheat flour
1 teaspoon grated orange peel, if desired
1½ cups fresh blueberries
1½ cups fresh raspberries
About 1 cup fat-free whipped cream topping (from aerosol can)

1 Heat oven to 375°F. In sandwich-size resealable food-storage plastic bag, combine 2 teaspoons sugar and ½ teaspoon of the cinnamon. Using cooking spray, spray both sides of tortilla, about 3 seconds per side; cut tortilla into 8 wedges. In bag with cinnamon-sugar, add wedges; seal bag. Shake to coat wedges evenly. 2. On ungreased cookie sheet, spread out wedges. Bake 7 to 9 minutes, turning once, until just beginning to crisp (wedges will continue to crisp while cooling). Cool about 15 minutes. 3. Meanwhile, spray 4 (6-ounce / 170-g) custard cups or ramekins with cooking spray; place cups on another cookie sheet. In small bowl, stir ¼ cup sugar, the flour, orange peel and remaining ¼ teaspoon cinnamon until blended. In medium bowl, gently toss berries with sugar mixture; divide evenly among custard cups. 4. Bake 15 minutes; stir gently. Bake 5 to 7 minutes longer or until liquid is bubbling around edges. Cool at least 15 minutes. 5. To serve, top each cup with about ¼ cup whipped cream topping; serve tortilla wedges with berry cups. Serve warm.

Per Serving
Calorie: 180 | fat: 2g | protein: 3g | carbs: 37g | sugars: 25g | fiber: 7g | sodium: 60mg

Berry Smoothie Pops

Prep time: 5 minutes | Cook time: 0 minutes | Serves 6

2 cups frozen mixed berries
1 cup plain nonfat Greek yogurt

½ cup unsweetened plain almond milk
2 tablespoons hemp seeds

1. Place all the ingredients in a blender and process until finely blended. 2. Pour into 6 clean ice pop molds and insert sticks. 3. Freeze for 3 to 4 hours until firm.

Per Serving

Calorie: 70 | fat: 2g | protein: 5g | carbs: 9g | sugars: 2g | fiber: 3g | sodium: 28mg

Instant Pot Tapioca

Prep time: 10 minutes | Cook time: 7 minutes | Serves 6

2 cups water
½ cup sugar
½ cup evaporated skim milk
1 teaspoon vanilla

1 cup small pearl tapioca
4 eggs
Sugar substitute to equal ¼ cup sugar
Fruit of choice, optional

1. Combine water and tapioca in Instant Pot. 2. Secure lid and make sure vent is set to sealing. Press Manual and set for 5 minutes. 3. Perform a quick release. Press Cancel, remove lid, and press Sauté. 4. Whisk together eggs and evaporated milk. SLOWLY add to the Instant Pot, stirring constantly so the eggs don't scramble. 5. Stir in the sugar substitute until it's dissolved, press Cancel, then stir in the vanilla. 6. Allow to cool thoroughly, then refrigerate at least 4 hours.

Per Serving

Calorie: 262 | fat: 3g | protein: 6g | carbs: 50g | sugars: 28g | fiber: 0g | sodium: 75mg

Oatmeal Cookies

Prep time: 5 minutes | Cook time: 15 minutes | Serves 16

¾ cup almond flour
¼ cup shredded unsweetened coconut
1 teaspoon ground cinnamon
¼ cup unsweetened applesauce
1 tablespoon pure maple syrup

¾ cup old-fashioned oats
1 teaspoon baking powder
¼ teaspoon salt
1 large egg
2 tablespoons coconut oil, melted

1. Preheat the oven to 350°F. 2. In a medium mixing bowl, combine the almond flour, oats, coconut, baking powder, cinnamon, and salt, and mix well. 3. In another medium bowl, combine the applesauce, egg, maple syrup, and coconut oil, and mix. Stir the wet mixture into the dry mixture. 4. Form the dough into balls a little bigger than a tablespoon and place on a baking sheet, leaving at least 1 inch between them. Bake for 12 minutes until the cookies are just browned. Remove from the oven and let cool for 5 minutes. 5. Using a spatula, remove the cookies and cool on a rack.

Per Serving

Calorie: 76 | fat: 6g | protein: 2g | carbs: 5g | sugars: 1g | fiber: 1g | sodium: 57mg

Raspberry Nice Cream

Prep time: 5 minutes | Cook time: 0 minutes | Serves 3

2 cups frozen, sliced, overripe bananas
2 cups frozen or fresh raspberries
Pinch of sea salt
1-2 tablespoons coconut nectar or 1-1½ tablespoons pure maple syrup

1. In a food processor or high-speed blender, combine the bananas, raspberries, salt, and 1 tablespoon of the nectar or syrup. Puree until smooth. Taste, and add the remaining nectar or syrup, if desired. Serve immediately, if you like a soft-serve consistency, or transfer to an airtight container and freeze for an hour or more, if you like a firmer texture.

Per Serving
Calorie: 193| fat: 1g | protein: 3g | carbs: 47g | sugars: 24g | fiber: 13g | sodium: 101mg

Chocolate Baked Bananas

Prep time: 10 minutes | Cook time: 8 to 10 minutes | Serves 5

4-5 large ripe bananas, sliced lengthwise
2 tablespoons coconut nectar or pure maple syrup
1 tablespoon cocoa powder
Couple pinches sea salt
2 tablespoons nondairy chocolate chips (for finishing)
1 tablespoon chopped pecans, walnuts, almonds, or pumpkin seeds (for finishing)

1. Line a baking sheet with parchment paper and preheat oven to 450°F. Place bananas on the parchment. In a bowl, mix the coconut nectar or maple syrup with the cocoa powder and salt. Stir well to fully combine. Drizzle the chocolate mixture over the bananas. 2. Bake for 8 to 10 minutes, until bananas are softened and caramelized. Sprinkle on chocolate chips and nuts, and serve.

Per Serving
Calorie: 146 | fat: 3g | protein: 2g | carbs: 34g | sugars: 18g | fiber: 4g | sodium: 119mg

Greek Yogurt Berry Smoothie Pops

Prep time: 5 minutes | Cook time: 0 minutes | Serves 6

2 cups frozen mixed berries
½ cup unsweetened plain almond milk
1 cup plain nonfat Greek yogurt
2 tablespoons hemp seeds

Place all the ingredients in a blender and process until finely blended.
Pour into 6 clean ice pop molds and insert sticks. 2. Freeze for 3 to 4 hours until firm.

Per Serving
calories: 70 | fat: 2g | protein: 5g | carbs: 9g | sugars: 2g | fiber: 3g | sodium: 28mg

Grilled Peach and Coconut Yogurt Bowls

Prep time: 5 minutes | Cook time: 10 minutes | Serves 4

2 peaches, halved and pitted
½ cup plain nonfat Greek yogurt
1 teaspoon pure vanilla extract
¼ cup unsweetened dried coconut flakes
2 tablespoons unsalted pistachios, shelled and broken into pieces

Preheat the broiler to high. Arrange the rack in the closest position to the broiler.
In a shallow pan, arrange the peach halves, cut-side up. Broil for 6 to 8 minutes until browned, tender, and hot. 2. In a small bowl, mix the yogurt and vanilla.
Spoon the yogurt into the cavity of each peach half. 3. Sprinkle 1 tablespoon of coconut flakes and 1½ teaspoons of pistachios over each peach half. Serve warm.

Per Serving
calories: 102 | fat: 5g | protein: 5g | carbs: 11g | sugars: 8g | fiber: 2g | sodium: 12mg

Frozen Chocolate Peanut Butter Bites

Prep time: 5 minutes | Cook time: 0 minutes | Serves 32

1 cup coconut oil, melted
¼ cup honey
¼ cup cocoa powder
¼ cup natural peanut butter

Pour the melted coconut oil into a medium bowl. Whisk in the cocoa powder, honey, and peanut butter. 2. Transfer the mixture to ice cube trays in portions about 1½ teaspoons each. 3. Freeze for 2 hours or until ready to serve.

Per Serving
calories: 80 | fat: 8g | protein: 1g | carbs: 3g | sugars: 2g | fiber: 0g | sodium: 20mg

Dark Chocolate Almond Butter Cups

Prep time: 15 minutes | Cook time: 0 minutes | Serves 12

½ cup natural almond butter
1 cup dark chocolate chips
1 tablespoon pure maple syrup
1 tablespoon coconut oil

Line a 12-cup muffin tin with cupcake liners. 2. In a medium bowl, mix the almond butter and maple syrup. If necessary, heat in the microwave to soften slightly. 3. Spoon about 2 teaspoons of the almond butter mixture into each muffin cup and press down to fill. 4. In a double boiler or the microwave, melt the chocolate chips. Stir in the coconut oil, and mix well to incorporate. 5. Drop 1 tablespoon of chocolate on top of each almond butter cup. 6. Freeze for at least 30 minutes to set. Thaw for 10 minutes before serving.

Per Serving
calories: 101 | fat: 8g | protein: 3g | carbs: 6g | sugars: 4g | fiber: 1g | sodium: 32mg

No-Bake Carrot Cake Bites

Prep time: 15 minutes | Cook time: 0 minutes | Serves 20

½ cup old-fashioned oats
6 dates, pitted
½ cup coconut flour
2 teaspoons pure maple syrup
½ teaspoon ground nutmeg

2 medium carrots, chopped
½ cup chopped walnuts
2 tablespoons hemp seeds
1 teaspoon ground cinnamon

In a blender jar, combine the oats and carrots, and process until finely ground. Transfer to a bowl. 2. Add the dates and walnuts to the blender and process until coarsely chopped. Return the oat-carrot mixture to the blender and add the coconut flour, hemp seeds, maple syrup, cinnamon, and nutmeg. Process until well mixed. 3. Using your hands, shape the dough into balls about the size of a tablespoon. 4. Store in the refrigerator in an airtight container for up to 1 week.

Per Serving

calories: 68 | fat: 3g | protein: 2g | carbs: 10g | sugars: 6g | fiber: 2g | sodium: 6mg

Ambrosia

Prep time: 10 minutes | Cook time: 0 minutes | Serves 8

3 oranges, peeled, sectioned, and quartered
1 cup shredded, unsweetened coconut

2 (4-ounce / 113-g) cups diced peaches in water, drained
1 (8-ounce / 227-g) container fat-free crème fraîche

In a large mixing bowl, combine the oranges, peaches, coconut, and crème fraîche. Gently toss until well mixed. Cover and refrigerate overnight.

Per Serving

calories: 111 | fat: 5g | protein: 2g | carbs: 12g | sugars: 8g | fiber: 3g | sodium: 7mg

Creamy Strawberry Crepes

Prep time: 10 minutes | Cook time: 10 minutes | Serves 4

½ cup old-fashioned oats
1 egg
Nonstick cooking spray
¼ cup low-fat cottage cheese

1 cup unsweetened plain almond milk
3 teaspoons honey, divided
2 ounces (57 g) low-fat cream cheese
2 cups sliced strawberries

In a blender jar, process the oats until they resemble flour. Add the almond milk, egg, and 1½ teaspoons honey, and process until smooth. 2. Heat a large skillet over medium heat. Spray with nonstick cooking spray to coat. 3. Add ¼ cup of oat batter to the pan and quickly swirl around to coat the bottom of the pan and let cook for 2 to 3 minutes. When the edges begin to turn brown, flip the crepe with a spatula and cook until lightly browned and firm, about 1 minute. Transfer to a plate. Continue with the remaining batter, spraying the skillet with nonstick cooking spray before adding more batter. Set the cooked crepes aside, loosely covered with aluminum foil, while you make the filling. 4. Clean the blender jar, then combine the cream cheese, cottage cheese, and remaining 1½ teaspoons honey, and process until smooth. 5. Fill each crepe with 2 tablespoons of the cream cheese mixture, topped with ¼ cup of strawberries. Serve.

Per Serving

calories: 149 | fat: 6g | protein: 6g | carbs: 20g | sugars: 10g | fiber: 3g | sodium: 177mg

Banana Pudding

Prep time: 30 minutes | Cook time: 20 minutes | Serves 10

Pudding:
¾ cup erythritol or other sugar replacement
¼ teaspoon salt
6 tablespoons prepared egg replacement
2 (8-ounce / 227-g) containers sugar-free spelt hazelnut biscuits, crushed
Meringue:
5 medium egg whites (1 cup)
½ teaspoon vanilla extract

5 teaspoons almond flour
2½ cups fat-free milk
½ teaspoon vanilla extract
5 medium bananas, sliced
5 medium bananas, sliced

¼ cup erythritol or other sugar replacement

Make the Pudding
In a saucepan, whisk the erythritol, almond flour, salt, and milk together. Cook over medium heat until the sugar is dissolved. 2. Whisk in the egg replacement and cook for about 10 minutes, or until thickened. 3. Remove from the heat and stir in the vanilla. 4. Spread the thickened pudding onto the bottom of a 3 × 6-inch casserole dish. 5. Arrange a layer of crushed biscuits on top of the pudding. 6. Place a layer of sliced bananas on top of the biscuits.
Make the Meringue
Preheat the oven to 350°F (180°C). 2. In a medium bowl, beat the egg whites for about 5 minutes, or until stiff. 3. Add the erythritol and vanilla while continuing to beat for about 3 more minutes. 4. Spread the meringue on top of the banana pudding. 5. Transfer the casserole dish to the oven, and bake for 7 to 10 minutes, or until the top is lightly browned.
Per Serving
calories: 323 | fat: 14g | protein: 12g | carbs: 42g | sugars: 11g | fiber: 3g | sodium: 148mg

Swirled Cream Cheese Brownies

Prep time: 10 minutes | Cook time: 20 minutes | Serves 12

2 eggs
¼ cup coconut oil, melted
¼ cup unsweetened cocoa powder
¼ teaspoon salt
2 tablespoons low-fat cream cheese

¼ cup unsweetened applesauce
3 tablespoons pure maple syrup, divided
¼ cup coconut flour
1 teaspoon baking powder

Preheat the oven to 350°F (180°C). Grease an 8-by-8-inch baking dish. 2. In a large mixing bowl, beat the eggs with the applesauce, coconut oil, and 2 tablespoons of maple syrup. 3. Stir in the cocoa powder and coconut flour, and mix well. Sprinkle the salt and baking powder evenly over the surface and mix well to incorporate. Transfer the mixture to the prepared baking dish. 4. In a small, microwave-safe bowl, microwave the cream cheese for 10 to 20 seconds until softened. Add the remaining 1 tablespoon of maple syrup and mix to combine. 5. Drop the cream cheese onto the batter, and use a toothpick or chopstick to swirl it on the surface. Bake for 20 minutes, until a toothpick inserted in the center comes out clean. Cool and cut into 12 squares. 6. Store refrigerated in a covered container for up to 5 days.
Per Serving
calories: 84 | fat: 6g | protein: 2g | carbs: 6g | sugars: 4g | fiber: 2g | sodium: 93mg

Maple Oatmeal Cookies

Prep time: 5 minutes | Cook time: 15 minutes | Serves 16

¾ cup almond flour
¼ cup shredded unsweetened coconut
1 teaspoon ground cinnamon
¼ cup unsweetened applesauce
1 tablespoon pure maple syrup

¾ cup old-fashioned oats
1 teaspoon baking powder
¼ teaspoon salt
1 large egg
2 tablespoons coconut oil, melted

Preheat the oven to 350°F (180°C). 2. In a medium mixing bowl, combine the almond flour, oats, coconut, baking powder, cinnamon, and salt, and mix well. 3. In another medium bowl, combine the applesauce, egg, maple syrup, and coconut oil, and mix. Stir the wet mixture into the dry mixture. 4. Form the dough into balls a little bigger than a tablespoon and place on a baking sheet, leaving at least 1 inch between them. Bake for 12 minutes until the cookies are just browned. Remove from the oven and let cool for 5 minutes. 5. Using a spatula, remove the cookies and cool on a rack.

Per Serving
calories: 76 | fat: 6g | protein: 2g | carbs: 5g | sugars: 1g | fiber: 1g | sodium: 57mg

Pineapple Nice Cream

Prep time: 10 minutes | Cook time: 0 minutes | Serves 6

2 cups frozen pineapple
½ cup unsweetened almond milk

1 cup peanut butter (no added sugar, salt, or fat)

In a blender or food processor, combine the frozen pineapple and peanut butter and process. 2. Add the almond milk, and blend until smooth. The end result should be a smooth paste.

Per Serving
calories: 301 | fat: 22g | protein: 14g | carbs: 15g | sugars: 8g | fiber: 4g | sodium: 39mg

Spiced Orange Rice Pudding

Prep time: 5 minutes | Cook time: 35 minutes | Serves 6

2 cups short-grain brown rice
1 teaspoon ground nutmeg, plus more for serving
¼ teaspoon orange extract
½ cup erythritol or other brown sugar replacement

6 cups fat-free milk
1 teaspoon ground cinnamon, plus more for serving
1 teaspoon ground cinnamon, plus more for serving
Juice of 2 oranges (about ¾ cup)

In an electric pressure cooker, stir the rice, milk, nutmeg, cinnamon, orange extract, orange juice, and erythritol together. 2. Close and lock the lid, and set the pressure valve to sealing. 3. Select the Manual setting, and cook for 35 minutes. 4. Once cooking is complete, quick-release the pressure. Carefully remove the lid. 5. Stir well and spoon into serving dishes. Enjoy with an additional sprinkle of nutmeg and cinnamon.

Per Serving
calories: 320 | fat: 2g | protein: 13g | carbs: 61g | sugars: 15g | fiber: 2g | sodium: 130mg

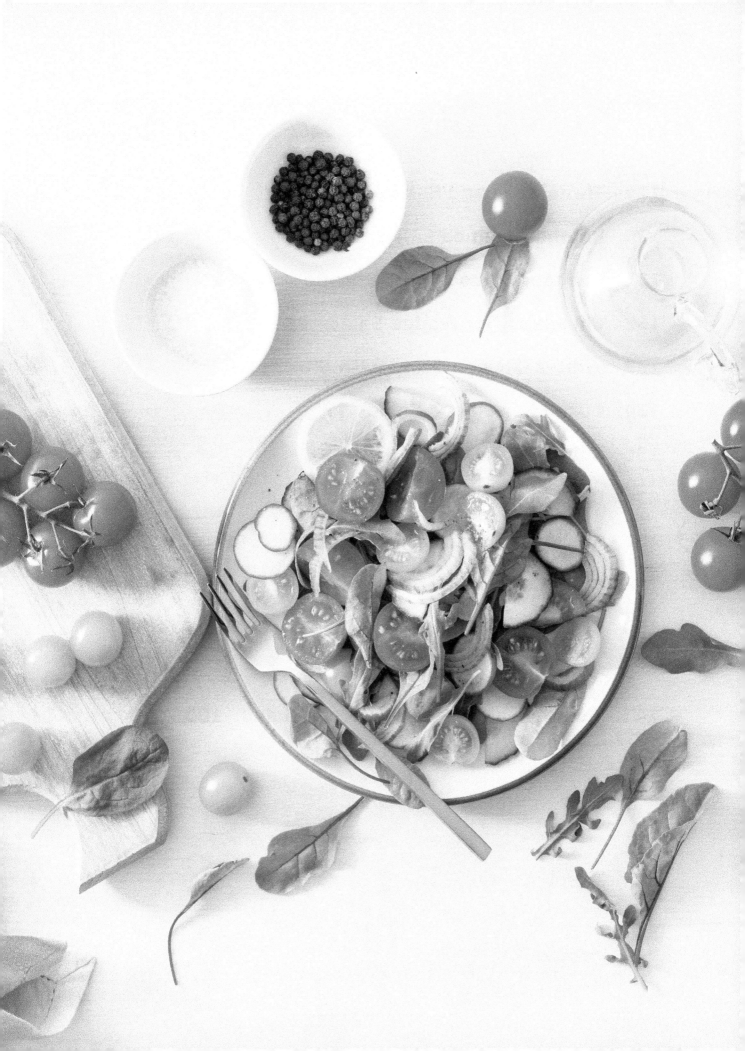

Chapter 11 Salads

Three Bean and Basil Salad

Prep time: 10 minutes | Cook time: 0 minutes | Serves 8

1 (15-ounce / 425-g) can low-sodium chickpeas, drained and rinsed
1 (15-ounce / 425-g) can low-sodium kidney beans, drained and rinsed
1 (15-ounce / 425-g) can low-sodium white beans, drained and rinsed
1 red bell pepper, seeded and finely chopped
¼ cup chopped scallions, both white and green parts
¼ cup finely chopped fresh basil
3 garlic cloves, minced
2 tablespoons extra-virgin olive oil
1 tablespoon red wine vinegar
1 teaspoon Dijon mustard
¼ teaspoon freshly ground black pepper

1. In a large mixing bowl, combine the chickpeas, kidney beans, white beans, bell pepper, scallions, basil, and garlic. Toss gently to combine. 2. In a small bowl, combine the olive oil, vinegar, mustard, and pepper. Toss with the salad. 3. Cover and refrigerate for an hour before serving, to allow the flavors to mix.

Per Serving
Calorie: 193 | fat: 5g | protein: 10g | carbs: 29g | sugars: 3g | fiber: 8g | sodium: 246mg

Rainbow Quinoa Salad

Prep time: 10 minutes | Cook time: 0 minutes | Serves 3

Dressing
3½ tablespoons orange juice
1 tablespoon pure maple syrup
Couple pinches of cloves
Freshly ground black pepper to taste

1 tablespoon apple cider vinegar
1½ teaspoons yellow mustard
Rounded ½ teaspoon sea salt

Salad
2 cups cooked quinoa, cooled
½ cup corn kernels
½ cup diced apple tossed in ½ teaspoon lemon juice
¼ cup diced red pepper
¼ cup sliced green onions or chives
1 can (15 ounces) black beans, rinsed and drained
Sea salt to taste
Freshly ground black pepper to taste

1. To make the dressing: In a large bowl, whisk together the orange juice, vinegar, syrup, mustard, cloves, salt, and pepper. 2. To make the salad: Add the quinoa, corn, apple, red pepper, green onion or chives, and black beans, and stir to combine well. Season with the salt and black pepper to taste. Serve, or store in an airtight container in the fridge.

Per Serving
Calorie: 355 | fat: 4g | protein: 15g | carbs: 68g | sugars: 12g | fiber: 15g | sodium: 955mg

Salmon, Quinoa, and Avocado Salad

Prep time: 15 minutes | Cook time: 20 minutes | Serves 4

½ cup quinoa
4 (4-ounce / 113-g) salmon fillets
1 teaspoon extra-virgin olive oil,
plus 2 tablespoons
½ teaspoon freshly ground black
pepper, divided
1 avocado, chopped
¼ cup chopped fresh cilantro
Juice of 1 lime

1 cup water
1 pound (454 g) asparagus, trimmed
½ teaspoon salt, divided
½ teaspoon salt, divided
¼ teaspoon red pepper flakes
¼ teaspoon red pepper flakes
¼ cup chopped scallions, both white and green parts
1 tablespoon minced fresh oregano

1. In a small pot, combine the quinoa and water, and bring to a boil over medium-high heat. Cover, reduce the heat, and simmer for 15 minutes. 2. Preheat the oven to 425°F. Line a large baking sheet with parchment paper. 3. Arrange the salmon on one side of the prepared baking sheet. Toss the asparagus with 1 teaspoon of olive oil, and arrange on the other side of the baking sheet. Season the salmon and asparagus with ¼ teaspoon of salt, ¼ teaspoon of pepper, and the red pepper flakes. Roast for 12 minutes until browned and cooked through. 4. While the fish and asparagus are cooking, in a large mixing bowl, gently toss the cooked quinoa, avocado, scallions, cilantro, and oregano. Add the remaining 2 tablespoons of olive oil and the lime juice, and season with the remaining ¼ teaspoon of salt and ¼ teaspoon of pepper. 5. Break the salmon into pieces, removing the skin and any bones, and chop the asparagus into bite-sized pieces. Fold into the quinoa and serve warm or at room temperature.

Per Serving
Calorie: 397 | fat: 22g | protein: 29g | carbs: 23g | sugars: 3g | fiber: 8g | sodium: 292mg

Cheeseburger Wedge Salad

Prep time: 15 minutes | Cook time: 10 minutes | Serves 4

salad
1 pound (454 g) lean ground beef
sliced in half lengthwise
½ cup (80 g) coarsely chopped tomatoes
1 small dill pickle, finely chopped (optional)

2 medium heads romaine lettuce, rinsed, dried, and
½ cup (60 g) shredded Cheddar cheese
⅓ cup (50 g) finely chopped red onion

dressing
2 ounces (57 g) no-salt-added tomato paste
2 tablespoons (30 ml) water
¼ teaspoon sea salt
¼ teaspoon garlic powder

2 tablespoons (30 ml) apple cider vinegar
1 tablespoon (15 ml) honey
½ teaspoon onion powder

1. To make the salad, heat a large skillet over medium-high heat. Once the skillet is hot, add the beef and cook it for 9 to 10 minutes, until it is brown and cooked though. 2. Meanwhile, place a ½ head of romaine lettuce on each of four plates. Divide the beef evenly on top of each of the romaine halves. Then top each with the Cheddar cheese, tomatoes, onion, and pickle (if using). 3. To make the dressing, combine the tomato paste, vinegar, water, honey, sea salt, onion powder, and garlic powder in a small mason jar, secure the lid on top, and shake the jar thoroughly until everything is combined. Drizzle the dressing evenly over each salad and serve.

Per Serving
Calorie: 320 | fat: 14g | protein: 32g | carbs: 19g | sugars: 11g | fiber: 8g | sodium: 341mg

Winter Chicken Salad with Citrus

Prep time: 10 minutes | Cook time: 0 minutes | Serves 4

4 cups baby spinach
1 tablespoon freshly squeezed lemon juice
Freshly ground black pepper, to taste
2 mandarin oranges, peeled and sectioned
¼ cup sliced almonds

2 tablespoons extra-virgin olive oil
⅛ teaspoon salt
2 cups chopped cooked chicken
½ peeled grapefruit, sectioned

In a large mixing bowl, toss the spinach with the olive oil, lemon juice, salt, and pepper. 2. Add the chicken, oranges, grapefruit, and almonds to the bowl. Toss gently. 3. Arrange on 4 plates and serve.

Per Serving
calories: 249 | fat: 12g | protein: 24g | carbs: 11g | sugars: 7g | fiber: 3g | sodium: 135mg

Cucumber-Mango Salad

Prep time: 20 minutes | Cook time: 0 minutes | Serves 4

1 small cucumber
¼ teaspoon grated lime peel
1 teaspoon honey
Pinch salt

1 medium mango
1 tablespoon lime juice
¼ teaspoon ground cumin
4 leaves Bibb lettuce

1 Cut cucumber lengthwise in half; scoop out seeds. Chop cucumber (about 1 cup). 2 Score skin of mango lengthwise into fourths with knife; peel skin. Cut peeled mango lengthwise close to both sides of pit. Chop mango into ½-inch cubes. 3. In small bowl, mix lime peel, lime juice, honey, cumin and salt. Stir in cucumber and mango. Place lettuce leaves on serving plates. Spoon mango mixture onto lettuce leaves.

Per Serving
Calorie: 50 | fat: 0g | protein: 0g | carbs: 12g | sugars: 9g | fiber: 1g | sodium: 40mg

Cabbage and Carrot Slaw

Prep time: 15 minutes | Cook time: 0 minutes | Serves 6

2 cups finely chopped green cabbage
2 cups grated carrots
2 tablespoons extra-virgin olive oil
1 teaspoon honey
¼ teaspoon salt

2 cups finely chopped red cabbage
3 scallions, both white and green parts, sliced
2 tablespoons rice vinegar
1 garlic clove, minced

In a large bowl, toss together the green and red cabbage, carrots, and scallions. 2. In a small bowl, whisk together the oil, vinegar, honey, garlic, and salt. 3. Pour the dressing over the veggies and mix to thoroughly combine. Serve immediately, or cover and chill for several hours before serving.

Per Serving
calories: 80 | fat: 5g | protein: 1g | carbs: 10g | sugars: 6g | fiber: 3g | sodium: 126mg

Blackberry Goat Cheese Salad

Prep time: 15 minutes | Cook time: 20 minutes | Serves 4

Vinaigrette:

1 pint blackberries

1 tablespoon honey

¼ teaspoon salt

2 tablespoons red wine vinegar

3 tablespoons extra-virgin olive oil

Freshly ground black pepper, to taste

Salad:

1 sweet potato, cubed

8 cups salad greens (baby spinach, spicy greens, romaine)

¼ cup crumbled goat cheese

1 teaspoon extra-virgin olive oil

½ red onion, sliced

½ red onion, sliced

Make the Vinaigrette

In a blender jar, combine the blackberries, vinegar, honey, oil, salt, and pepper, and process until smooth. Set aside.

Make the Salad

Preheat the oven to 425ºF (220ºC). Line a baking sheet with parchment paper. 2. In a medium mixing bowl, toss the sweet potato with the olive oil. Transfer to the prepared baking sheet and roast for 20 minutes, stirring once halfway through, until tender. Remove and cool for a few minutes. 3. In a large bowl, toss the greens with the red onion and cooled sweet potato, and drizzle with the vinaigrette. Serve topped with 1 tablespoon of goat cheese per serving.

Per Serving

calories: 196 | fat: 12g | protein: 3g | carbs: 21g | sugars: 10g | fiber: 6g | sodium: 184mg

Garlic and Basil Three Bean Salad

Prep time: 10 minutes | Cook time: 0 minutes | Serves 8

1 (15-ounce / 425-g) can low-sodium chickpeas, drained and rinsed

1 (15-ounce / 425-g) can low-sodium kidney beans, drained and rinsed

1 (15-ounce / 425-g) can low-sodium white beans, drained and rinsed

1 red bell pepper, seeded and finely chopped

¼ cup chopped scallions, both white and green parts

¼ cup finely chopped fresh basil

3 garlic cloves, minced

2 tablespoons extra-virgin olive oil

1 tablespoon red wine vinegar

1 teaspoon Dijon mustard

¼ teaspoon freshly ground black pepper

In a large mixing bowl, combine the chickpeas, kidney beans, white beans, bell pepper, scallions, basil, and garlic. Toss gently to combine. 2. In a small bowl, combine the olive oil, vinegar, mustard, and pepper. Toss with the salad. 3. Cover and refrigerate for an hour before serving, to allow the flavors to mix.

Per Serving

calories: 193 | fat: 5g | protein: 10g | carbs: 29g | sugars: 3g | fiber: 8g | sodium: 246mg

Rainbow Black Bean Salad

Prep time: 15 minutes | Cook time: 0 minutes | Serves 5

1 (15-ounce / 425-g) can low-sodium
black beans, drained and rinsed
1 cup cherry
1 cup chopped baby spinach
¼ cup finely chopped jicama
¼ cup chopped fresh cilantro
1 tablespoon extra-virgin olive oil
1 teaspoon honey
¼ teaspoon freshly ground black pepper

1 avocado, diced
1 avocado, diced
tomatoes, halved
½ cup finely chopped red bell pepper
½ cup chopped scallions, both white and green parts
2 tablespoons freshly squeezed lime juice
2 garlic cloves, minced
¼ teaspoon salt

In a large bowl, combine the black beans, avocado, tomatoes, spinach, bell pepper, jicama, scallions, and cilantro. 2. In a small bowl, mix the lime juice, oil, garlic, honey, salt, and pepper. Add to the salad and toss. 3. Chill for 1 hour before serving.

Per Serving

calories: 169 | fat: 7g | protein: 6g | carbs: 22g | sugars: 3g | fiber: 9g | sodium: 235mg

Squash and Barley Salad

Prep time: 20 minutes | Cook time: 40 minutes | Serves 8

1 small butternut squash
extra-virgin olive oil, divided
1 cup pearl barley
2 cups baby kale
2 tablespoons balsamic vinegar
½ teaspoon salt

3 teaspoons plus 2 tablespoons
2 cups broccoli florets
1 cup toasted chopped walnuts
½ red onion, sliced
2 garlic cloves, minced
¼ teaspoon freshly ground black pepper

Preheat the oven to 400°F (205°C). Line a baking sheet with parchment paper. 2. Peel and seed the squash, and cut it into dice. In a large bowl, toss the squash with 2 teaspoons of olive oil. Transfer to the prepared baking sheet and roast for 20 minutes. 3. While the squash is roasting, toss the broccoli in the same bowl with 1 teaspoon of olive oil. After 20 minutes, flip the squash and push it to one side of the baking sheet. Add the broccoli to the other side and continue to roast for 20 more minutes until tender. 4. While the veggies are roasting, in a medium pot, cover the barley with several inches of water. Bring to a boil, then reduce the heat, cover, and simmer for 30 minutes until tender. Drain and rinse. 5. Transfer the barley to a large bowl, and toss with the cooked squash and broccoli, walnuts, kale, and onion. 6. In a small bowl, mix the remaining 2 tablespoons of olive oil, balsamic vinegar, garlic, salt, and pepper. Toss the salad with the dressing and serve.

Per Serving

calories: 275 | fat: 15g | protein: 6g | carbs: 32g | sugars: 3g | fiber: 7g | sodium: 144mg

Blueberry Chicken Salad

Prep time: 10 minutes | Cook time: 0 minutes | Serves 4

2 cups chopped cooked chicken
¼ cup finely chopped almonds
¼ cup finely chopped red onion
1 tablespoon chopped fresh cilantro
¼ teaspoon salt
8 cups salad greens (baby spinach, spicy greens, romaine)

1 cup fresh blueberries
1 celery stalk, finely chopped
1 tablespoon chopped fresh basil
½ cup plain, nonfat Greek yogurt or vegan mayonnaise
¼ teaspoon freshly ground black pepper

In a large mixing bowl, combine the chicken, blueberries, almonds, celery, onion, basil, and cilantro. Toss gently to mix. 2. In a small bowl, combine the yogurt, salt, and pepper. Add to the chicken salad and stir to combine.

Arrange 2 cups of salad greens on each of 4 plates and divide the chicken salad among the plates to serve.

Per Serving

calories: 207 | fat: 6g | protein: 28g | carbs: 11g | sugars: 6g | fiber: 3g | sodium: 235mg

Quinoa, Salmon, and Avocado Salad

Prep time: 15 minutes | Cook time: 20 minutes | Serves 4

½ cup quinoa
4 (4-ounce / 113-g) salmon fillets
1 teaspoon extra-virgin olive oil,
plus 2 tablespoons
½ teaspoon freshly ground
black pepper, divided
¼ teaspoon red pepper flakes
¼ cup chopped scallions, both
white and green parts
1 tablespoon minced fresh oregano

1 cup water
1 pound (454 g) asparagus, trimmed
½ teaspoon salt, divided
½ teaspoon salt, divided
¼ teaspoon red pepper flakes
¼ teaspoon red pepper flakes
1 avocado, chopped
¼ cup chopped fresh cilantro
¼ cup chopped fresh cilantro
Juice of 1 lime

1. In a small pot, combine the quinoa and water, and bring to a boil over medium-high heat. Cover, reduce the heat, and simmer for 15 minutes. 2. Preheat the oven to 425°F (220°C). Line a large baking sheet with parchment paper.Arrange the salmon on one side of the prepared baking sheet. Toss the asparagus with 1 teaspoon of olive oil, and arrange on the other side of the baking sheet. Season the salmon and asparagus with ¼ teaspoon of salt, ¼ teaspoon of pepper, and the red pepper flakes. Roast for 12 minutes until browned and cooked through. 3. While the fish and asparagus are cooking, in a large mixing bowl, gently toss the cooked quinoa, avocado, scallions, cilantro, and oregano. Add the remaining 2 tablespoons of olive oil and the lime juice, and season with the remaining ¼ teaspoon of salt and ¼ teaspoon of pepper. 4. Break the salmon into pieces, removing the skin and any bones, and chop the asparagus into bite-sized pieces. Fold into the quinoa and serve warm or at room temperature.

Per Serving

calories: 397 | fat: 22g | protein: 29g | carbs: 23g | sugars: 3g | fiber: 8g | sodium: 292mg

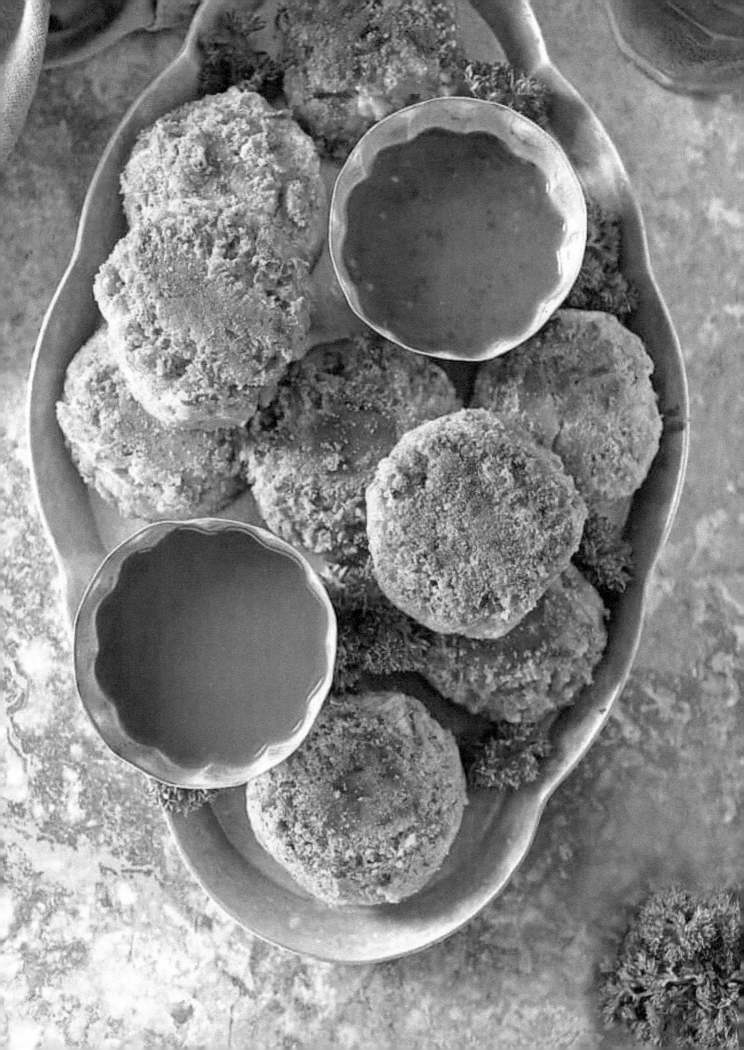

Chapter 12 Staples, Sauces, Dips, and Dressings

Caramelized Onion and Greek Yogurt Dip

Prep time: 10 minutes | Cook time: 45 minutes | Serves 8

2 tablespoons extra-virgin olive oil
1 garlic clove, minced
1 teaspoon salt

3 cups chopped onions
2 cups plain nonfat Greek yogurt
Freshly ground black pepper

1. In a large pot, heat the olive oil over medium heat until shimmering. Add the onions, and stir well to coat. Reduce heat to low, cover, and cook for 45 minutes, stirring every the 5 to 10 minutes, until well-browned and caramelized. Add the garlic and stir until just fragrant. 2. Remove from the heat and let cool for 10 minutes. 3. In a mixing bowl, combine the onions, yogurt, salt, and pepper.
Per Serving
Calorie: 83 | fat: 4g | protein: 6g | carbs: 7g | sugars: 5g | fiber: 1g | sodium: 264mg

Lime Zinger Dressing

Prep time: 5 minutes | Cook time: 0 minutes | Serves 4

¼ cup freshly squeezed lime juice
½ tablespoon ground chia seeds
½ teaspoon ground cumin
Pinch of allspice
Freshly ground black pepper to taste

3 tablespoons coconut nectar
½ tablespoon Dijon mustard
¼ teaspoon cinnamon
½ teaspoon sea salt
1 tablespoon water (optional)

1. In a blender, combine the lime juice, nectar, chia seeds, mustard, cumin, cinnamon, allspice, salt, and pepper. Puree until smooth. 2. Add the water if desired to thin. Transfer to a jar or other airtight container and refrigerate for up to a week.
Per Serving
Calorie: 52 | fat: 1g | protein: 0g | carbs: 12g | sugars: 9g | fiber: 1g | sodium: 340mg

Avocado Basil Dressing

Prep time: 5 minutes | Cook time: 0 minutes | Serves 6

¾ cup cubed ripe avocado (about 1 medium avocado)
1½ tablespoons freshly squeezed lemon juice
¼ cup loosely packed fresh basil leaves
Rounded ¼ teaspoon sea salt
Freshly ground black pepper to taste
½ cup + 1-2 tablespoons water
1-1½ teaspoons coconut nectar or pure maple syrup

1. In a blender, combine the avocado, lemon juice, basil, salt, pepper, ½ cup of the water, and 1 teaspoon of the nectar or syrup. Puree until very smooth. Add the additional 1 to 2 tablespoons water to thin to the desired consistency and the additional ½ teaspoon of nectar or syrup, if desired. Season with additional salt and pepper to taste.
Per Serving
Calorie: 41 | fat: 3g | protein: 0g | carbs: 4g | sugars: 2g | fiber: 1g | sodium: 149mg

Green Chickpea Hummus

Prep time: 5 minutes | Cook time: 0 minutes | Serves 6

2 cups frozen green chickpeas
¼ cup lemon juice
⅓ cup fresh basil leaves
1 tablespoon tahini
½ teaspoon ground cumin
½ teaspoon lemon zest (optional)

1 can (15 ounces) white beans, rinsed and drained
1 large clove garlic (or more to taste)
⅓ cup fresh parsley leaves
1 teaspoon sea salt
1-2 tablespoons water (optional)

Add the chickpeas to a pot of boiling water and cook for just a minute to bring out their vibrant green color. Remove, run under cold water to stop the cooking process, and drain. In a food processor, combine the chickpeas, beans, lemon juice, garlic, basil, parsley, tahini, salt, and cumin. 2. Puree until smooth, scraping down the bowl as needed. Add the water if desired to thin or help the pureeing process. Add the lemon zest, if desired, and season to taste. Serve.

Per Serving
Calorie: 176 | fat: 3g | protein: 10g | carbs: 29g | sugars: 3g | fiber: 8g | sodium: 477mg

Punchy Mustard Vinaigrette

Prep time: 5 minutes | Cook time: 0 minutes | Serves 6

¼ cup apple cider vinegar or rice vinegar
1½ tablespoons yellow or Dijon mustard
½ tablespoon ground chia
⅛ teaspoon sea salt

2 tablespoons tamari
2½ tablespoons coconut nectar or pure maple syrup
Freshly ground black pepper to taste

1. In a blender, combine the vinegar, tamari, mustard, nectar or syrup, chia, pepper, and salt. Puree until fully incorporated. Taste, and add extra mustard if you love it! Season to taste with additional salt and pepper, if desired. 2. Serve immediately or refrigerate. Dressing will keep for at least a week in the fridge.

Per Serving
Calorie: 33 | fat: 0g | protein: 1g | carbs: 7g | sugars: 5g | fiber: 1g | sodium: 428mg

Dreamy Caesar Dressing

Prep time: 10 minutes | Cook time: 0 minutes | Serves 12

¼-⅓ cup soaked almonds or cashews
2 tablespoons freshly squeezed lemon juice
1 medium or large clove garlic, chopped (adjust to taste)
1 tablespoon chickpea miso (or other mild-flavored miso)
2 teaspoons Dijon mustard
Freshly ground black pepper to taste
1 teaspoon pure maple syrup
¾ cup plain low-fat nondairy milk
2-3 tablespoons water or nondairy milk (optional)

½ cup cooked red or yellow potato, skins removed
1½ tablespoons red wine vinegar

½ teaspoon sea salt

1. In a blender, combine the nuts, potato, lemon juice, vinegar, garlic, miso, mustard, salt, pepper, syrup, and milk. Puree until very smooth. Add the water or additional milk to thin the dressing, if desired. (It will thicken after refrigeration.)

Per Serving

Calorie: 34 | fat: 2g | protein: 1g | carbs: 4g | sugars: 1g | fiber: 1g | sodium: 177mg

Fresh Salsa

Prep time: 10 minutes | Cook time: 0 minutes | Serves 4

2 cups chopped tomatoes

¼ cup minced onion or ⅓ cup chopped green onion

¼ cup minced red, yellow, or orange bell pepper

1 small jalapeño pepper, seeded and minced, wear plastic gloves when handling

1 large clove garlic, minced or grated

1 tablespoon lime juice

½ teaspoon sea salt

½ teaspoon cumin (optional)

⅛ teaspoon allspice

Freshly ground black pepper to taste

¼ cup minced cilantro (optional)

In a large bowl, combine the tomatoes, onion, bell pepper, jalapeño pepper, garlic, lime juice, salt, cumin (if using), allspice, black pepper, and cilantro (if using). Stir to combine. 2. Taste, and add extra salt or spices as desired. Serve or refrigerate in an airtight container until ready to use (within 2 to 3 days).

Per Serving

Calorie: 27 | fat: 0g | protein: 1g | carbs: 6g | sugars: 3g | fiber: 2g | sodium: 301mg

Fresh Tomato Salsa

Prep time: 10 minutes | Cook time: 0 minutes | Serves 6

2 or 3 medium, ripe tomatoes, diced

½ red onion, minced

1 serrano pepper, seeded and minced

Juice of 1 lime

¼ cup minced fresh cilantro

¼ teaspoon salt

1. In a small bowl, combine the tomatoes, onion, serrano pepper, lime juice, cilantro, and salt, and mix well. Taste and season with additional salt as needed. 2. Serve immediately, or transfer to an airtight container and refrigerate for up to 3 days.

Per Serving

Calorie: 18 | fat: 0g | protein: 1g | carbs: 4g | sugars: 1g | fiber: 1g | sodium: 84mg

Oregano Tomato Marinara

Prep time: 5 minutes | Cook time: 15 minutes | Serves 8

1 (28-ounce / 794-g) can whole tomatoes
2 tablespoons extra-virgin olive oil
4 garlic cloves, minced
½ teaspoon salt
¼ teaspoon dried oregano

Discard about half of the liquid from the can of tomatoes, and transfer the tomatoes and remaining liquid to a large bowl. Use clean hands or a large spoon to break the tomatoes apart. 2. In a large skillet, heat the olive oil over medium heat. Add the garlic and salt, and cook until the garlic just begins to sizzle, without letting it brown. 3. Add the tomatoes and their liquid to the skillet. 4. Simmer the sauce for about 15 minutes until the oil begins to separate and become dark orange and the sauce thickens. Add the oregano, stir, and remove from the heat. 5. After the marinara has cooled to room temperature, store in glass containers in the refrigerator for up to 3 or 4 days, or in zip-top freezer bags for up to 4 months.
Per Serving
calories: 48 | fat: 4g | protein: 1g | carbs: 4g | sugars: 2g | fiber: 1g | sodium: 145mg

Lime Tomato Salsa

Prep time: 10 minutes | Cook time: 0 minutes | Serves 6

2 or 3 medium, ripe tomatoes, diced
½ red onion, minced
1 serrano pepper, seeded and minced
Juice of 1 lime
¼ cup minced fresh cilantro
¼ teaspoon salt

In a small bowl, combine the tomatoes, onion, serrano pepper, lime juice, cilantro, and salt, and mix well. Taste and season with additional salt as needed. 2. Serve immediately, or transfer to an airtight container and refrigerate for up to 3 days.
Per Serving
calories: 18 | fat: 0g | protein: 1g | carbs: 4g | sugars: 1g | fiber: 1g | sodium: 84mg

Conclusion

Many curious friends have asked me, "did the recipes and lifestyle recommendation you complied in the Type 2 Diabetes Cookbook for Beginners reverse your diabetes?" I tell them, "absolutely." They become more eager, and then they ask again, "Did I cure it?" I tell them, "Not yet. However, I have lost over 6 kg and have a longer track record of normal blood glucose levels. I have no desire or need to go back to my old habits of unhealthy eating." I may try a delicious-looking sweet pastry at my favorite cafe down the street and see what happens. I don't think a little treat will hurt anyone. That's the edge Type 2 diabetes cookbook for beginners has over every other diabetes cookbook. The freedom to eat healthy foods while also eating the best. Coming up with a healthy diabetic diet doesn't have to be mind-boggling, and you don't have to let go of all your favorite foods because you're diabetic. The first step to making healthy and smarter choices is to make lifestyle changes through a healthy diet, healthy living and exercising. As with any healthy eating plan, a diabetic diet is more about the overall dietary pattern rather than obsessing over specific foods. Follow the 21-day meal plan in this book and eat more natural, unprocessed food and less packaged and convenient foods to enjoy good health.

Appendix 1 Measurement Conversion Chart

VOLUME EQUIVALENTS(DRY)

US STANDARD	METRIC (APPROXIMATE)
1/8 teaspoon	0.5 mL
1/4 teaspoon	1 mL
1/2 teaspoon	2 mL
3/4 teaspoon	4 mL
1 teaspoon	5 mL
1 tablespoon	15 mL
1/4 cup	59 mL
1/2 cup	118 mL
3/4 cup	177 mL
1 cup	235 mL
2 cups	475 mL
3 cups	700 mL
4 cups	1 L

VOLUME EQUIVALENTS(LIQUID)

US STANDARD	US STANDARD (OUNCES)	METRIC (APPROXIMATE)
2 tablespoons	1 fl.oz.	30 mL
1/4 cup	2 fl.oz.	60 mL
1/2 cup	4 fl.oz.	120 mL
1 cup	8 fl.oz.	240 mL
1 1/2 cup	12 fl.oz.	355 mL
2 cups or 1 pint	16 fl.oz.	475 mL
4 cups or 1 quart	32 fl.oz.	1 L
1 gallon	128 fl.oz.	4 L

TEMPERATURES EQUIVALENTS

FAHRENHEIT(F)	CELSIUS(C) (APPROXIMATE)
225 °F	107 °C
250 °F	120 °C
275 °F	135 °C
300 °F	150 °C
325 °F	160 °C
350 °F	180 °C
375 °F	190 °C
400 °F	205 °C
425 °F	220 °C
450 °F	235 °C
475 °F	245 °C
500 °F	260 °C

WEIGHT EQUIVALENTS

US STANDARD	METRIC (APPROXIMATE)
1 ounce	28 g
2 ounces	57 g
5 ounces	142 g
10 ounces	284 g
15 ounces	425 g
16 ounces (1 pound)	455 g
1.5 pounds	680 g
2 pounds	907 g

Appendix 2 The Dirty Dozen and Clean Fifteen

The Environmental Working Group (EWG) is a nonprofit, nonpartisan organization dedicated to protecting human health and the environment Its mission is to empower people to live healthier lives in a healthier environment. This organization publishes an annual list of the twelve kinds of produce, in sequence, that have the highest amount of pesticide residue-the Dirty Dozen-as well as a list of the fifteen kinds ofproduce that have the least amount of pesticide residue-the Clean Fifteen.

THE DIRTY DOZEN

- The 2016 Dirty Dozen includes the following produce. These are considered among the year's most important produce to buy organic:

Strawberries	Spinach
Apples	Tomatoes
Nectarines	Bell peppers
Peaches	Cherry tomatoes
Celery	Cucumbers
Grapes	Kale/collard greens
Cherries	Hot peppers

- *The Dirty Dozen list contains two additional itemskale/collard greens and hot peppers-because they tend to contain trace levels of highly hazardous pesticides.*

THE CLEAN FIFTEEN

- The least critical to buy organically are the Clean Fifteen list. The following are on the 2016 list:

Avocados	Papayas
Corn	Kiw
Pineapples	Eggplant
Cabbage	Honeydew
Sweet peas	Grapefruit
Onions	Cantaloupe
Asparagus	Cauliflower
Mangos	

- *Some of the sweet corn sold in the United States are made from genetically engineered (GE) seedstock. Buy organic varieties of these crops to avoid GE produce.*

CPSIA information can be obtained
at www.ICGtesting.com
Printed in the USA
BVHW090555040921
615986BV00010B/735